Clinics in
Gastroenterology

Hepatobiliary and Pancreatic Disorders

Clinics in
Gastroenterology

Hepatobiliary and Pancreatic Disorders

Alaka K Deshpande MD, MNAMS, FIMSA, FICP

Padmashree Awardee (2001) for Medical Services

Former Professor and Head
Department of Medicine
Grant Medical College and Sir JJ Group of Hospitals
Mumbai
Maharashtra, India

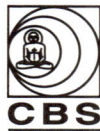

CBS

CBS Publishers & Distributors Pvt Ltd

New Delhi • Bengaluru • Chennai • Kochi • Kolkata • Mumbai
Hyderabad • Jharkhand • Nagpur • Patna • Pune • Uttarakhand

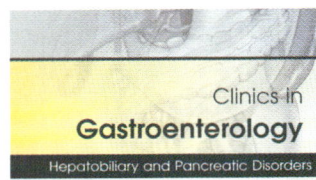

Clinics in
Gastroenterology
Hepatobiliary and Pancreatic Disorders

ISBN: 978-93-86478-13-9

Copyright © Author and Publisher

First Edition: 2018

Published by Satish Kumar Jain and produced by Varun Jain for

CBS Publishers & Distributors Pvt Ltd

4819/XI Prahlad Street, 24 Ansari Road, Daryaganj, New Delhi 110 002, India.

Ph: 23289259, 23266861, 23266867   Website: www.cbspd.com

Fax: 011-23243014   e-mail: delhi@cbspd.com; cbspubs@airtelmail.in.

Corporate Office: 204 FIE, Industrial Area, Patparganj, Delhi 110 092

Ph: 4934 4934   Fax: 4934 4935   e-mail: publishing@cbspd.com; publicity@cbspd.com

Branches

- **Bengaluru:** Seema House 2975, 17th Cross, K.R. Road,
  Banasankari 2nd Stage, Bengaluru 560 070, Karnataka
  Ph: +91-80-26771678/79   Fax: +91-80-26771680   e-mail: bangalore@cbspd.com
- **Chennai:** 7, Subbaraya Street, Shenoy Nagar, Chennai 600 030, Tamil Nadu
  Ph: +91-44-26680620, 26681266   Fax: +91-44-42032115   e-mail: chennai@cbspd.com
- **Kochi:** Ashana House, No. 39/1904, AM Thomas Road, Valanjambalam,
  Ernakulam 682 016, Kochi, Kerala
  Ph: +91-484-4059061-62-64-65   Fax: +91-484-4059065   e-mail: kochi@cbspd.com
- **Kolkata:** 6/B, Ground Floor, Rameswar Shaw Road, Kolkata-700 014, West Bengal
  Ph: +91-33-22891126, 22891127, 22891128   e-mail: kolkata@cbspd.com
- **Mumbai:** 83-C, Dr E Moses Road, Worli, Mumbai-400018, Maharashtra
  Ph: +91-22-24902340/41   Fax: +91-22-24902342   e-mail: mumbai@cbspd.com

Representatives

- **Hyderabad** 0-9885175004   • **Jharkhand** 0-9811541605   • **Nagpur** 0-9021734563
- **Patna** 0-9334159340   • **Pune** 0-9623451994   • **Uttarakhand** 0-9716462459

Printed at International Print-O-Pac Limited, Noida, UP, India

Foreword

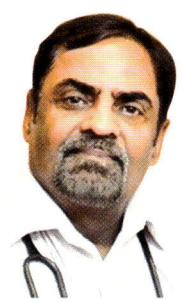

Clinics in Gastroenterology: Hepatobiliary and Pancreatic Disorders authored by Dr Alaka K Deshpande is a comprehensive text for the undergraduate students. It provides a wonderful insight to the students, giving them clinical perspectives of virtually all the aspects of hepatobiliary and pancreatic disorders. The language is simple and ably guides the students on each of the topics providing the information to the reader in an easy to comprehend manner.

Although the text is meant for undergraduate students, it undoubtedly provides a valuable read for even postgraduate students, since it provides up-to-date information on each subject of discussion like the application of fibroscan and serum ammonia levels, to name a few. The book contains clinically relevant topics like 'splenomegaly', dwelling on the extra-gastroenterological causes as well in the book. Subjects which have been increasingly gaining importance in recent times like 'non-alcoholic fatty liver disease' and 'liver transplantation' have been adequately discussed, in addition to topics like 'liver in pregnancy' and 'HIV disease and liver', which are not discussed in most texts.

There are numerous diagrams, flowcharts and tables which catch the attention of the reader and break the monotony of reading long texts; such a vital aspect for the success of any book. Another noteworthy feature is that the causes, clinical features and management guidelines are mentioned point-wise, providing the students an opportunity to use this book as a ready-reckoner in the out-patient clinics, emergency rooms and wards. This succinct text is not voluminous and will justify its launch as a handbook on such an important topic of hepatobiliary and pancreatic disorders.

I will also like to pen a couple of words about Dr Alaka K Deshpande, who is a celebrated teacher, practitioner and researcher, and a very senior and experienced physician of national repute. She deserves accolades for having decided to put her vast clinical experience in words through the medium of this book to benefit the present and future generations of medical students.

I wish the book and its author Dr Alaka K Deshpande a great success.

Rajesh Upadhyay
Director and Head
Department of Gastroenterology and Hepatology
Max Super-Speciality Hospital
Shalimar Bagh, Delhi
BC Roy Award, 2017
President, Association of Physicians of India, 2015

Preface

Hepatopancreatic disorders are common in the practice of internal medicine, ranging from asymptomatic rise in enzyme to fatal complications necessitating liver transplantation.

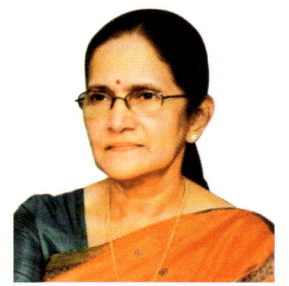

The liver is the largest organ in the human body carrying out various functions like large industry. It makes liver most vulnerable to various insults resulting into hepatic dysfunction which affects other body systems.

This is a clinical handbook to facilitate the bedside evaluation of the patient with hepatopancreatic disorders. It is designed to give organized clinical approach starting with anatomy, physiology, pathogenesis of the disorder, clinical features to arrive at a diagnosis followed by relevant investigations and management. The illustrations are self-explanatory. The language is simple used for bedside clinics.

Although liver has a tremendous capacity to regenerate, a large number of patients with severe structural damage to the liver require liver transplantation. The book has one full chapter on liver transplant.

With advances in imaging techniques and interventions, the pancreatic disorders are being diagnosed and managed successfully.

The experts in the field with their wisdom and experience have made a significant contribution to this handbook. I am thankful to all of them for their cooperation and contribution.

My students have inspired me to write and hence I dedicate the book to my students and my patients.

Finally, I am grateful to Mr SK Jain (CMD), Mr Varun Jain (Director), Mr YN Arjuna (Sr VP– Publishing), and Mr Ramesh Krishnamachari of CBS Publishers & Distributors, New Delhi, for putting in a great deal of efforts to bring out the book in a given time.

Alaka K Deshpande
MD, MAMS, FIMSA, FICP

Consultant Physician
Former Professor and Head
Department of Medicine
Grant Medical College & Sir JJ Group of Hospitals
Mumbai

Contributors

Alaka K Deshpande MD, MNAMS, FIMSA, FICP
Consultant Physician
Former Professor and Head, Department of Medicine, Grant Medical College and Sir JJ Group of Hospitals
Mumbai

Deepak Amarapurkar MD, DM, FACG, FICP, AGFA and FAASLD
Consultant Gastroenterologist, Bombay Hospital and Medical Research Centre
Breach Candy Hospital
Mumbai

Nirav Pipaliya MD, DM
Senior Registrar
Department of Gastroenterology
Lokmanya Tilak Municipal Medical College and General Hospital
Mumbai

Prabha Sawant MD, DM
Professor and Head
Department of Gastroenterology
Lokmanya Tilak Municipal
Medical College and
General Hospital
Mumbai

Pratibha Balasaheb MD, MED, DNB
Ex-Registrar, Bombay Hospital, Mumbai
Assistant Lecturer, Vasantrao Pawar Medical College, Nashik
Consultant Gastroenterologist and Hepatologist, KARE Clinic
Nashik

Ravi Mohanka MBBS, MS (Surgery),
DNB (Surgery), ASTS Fellowship (Transplant Surgery),
IAGES Fellowship (Advanced Laparoscic HPB Surgery)
Chief Surgeon and Head, Department of Liver Transplant Surgery, Global Hospital
Mumbai

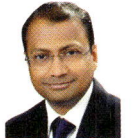

Samir Shah MD, DM (Gastro)
Head, Department of Hepatology Institute of Liver Diseases, HPB Surgery and Transplant, Global Hospital Mumbai, and Visiting Consultant Jaslok Hospital and Research Centre and Breach Candy Hospital, Mumbai

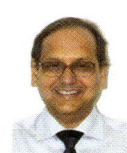

Shamsher Singh Chauhan MD (Med)
Fellow in Gastroenterology
LTMMGH, Sion, Mumbai

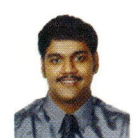

Somnath Chattopadhyay
MS (Gen Surg), DNB (Gen Surg), DNB (Surgical Gastroenterology), ASTS Fellow (American College of Transplant Surgeons) (Multiorgan Abdominal Transplant Surgery)
Consultant, Hepato-pancreato- biliary (HPB) and Transplant Surgery, Global Hospitals, Mumbai

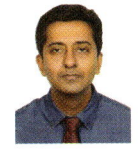

Upasna Bahure MS (Gen. Surg.)
Fellow in HPB and Transplant Surgery
Global Hospital, Mumbai

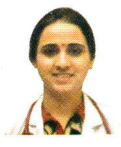

Viral Patrawala MD (Med) DM (Gastro)
Consultant in Gastroenterology
LH Hiranandani Hospital and Res Centre Powai, and Godrej Hospital, Vikroli
Mumbai

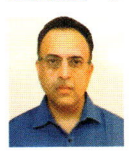

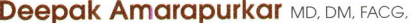

Contents

General Consideration in Hepatobiliary Diseases

Alaka Deshpande

A. LIVER ANATOMY AND FUNCTIONS

The liver is the largest organ in the body located in the right upper quadrant of the abdomen sheltered by the ribs. The upper border lies approximately at the level of the nipples. Normally, the liver dullness on percussion starts in the right fifth intercostal space in the mid-clavicular line.

The liver weighs about 1200–1500 grams. It has two lobes right and the left separated anteriorly by a peritoneal fold called as falcifarm ligament, posteriorly by the fissure for the ligamentum venosum, and inferiorly by the fissure for the ligamentum teres (Fig. 1.1).

It receives blood supply approximately two-thirds of which comes from the portal vein and about one-third from the hepatic artery which originates from the celiac axis. These vessels enter the liver through a fissure, porta hepatis situated on the inferior surface. Inside the liver these vessels break into right and left branches.

The venous drainage of the liver is by right and left hepatic veins which emerge from the back of the liver and at once, join inferior vena cava near its point of entry into the right atrium.

The basic morphological unit of the liver is a lobule in which a terminal radical of the hepatic vein is located at the centre and at the periphery is the portal triad consisting of terminal branch of hepatic artery, a portal vein, and a bile duct.

There is a uniform arrangement of portal triads separated by liver parenchyma composed of hepatocellular plates and sinusoids. Hepatocytes comprise of 65% of cells in the liver and 80% of the liver volume.

They are arranged in plates of one cell thickness radiating from the central vein to the periphery. In between the plates are the blood filled sinusoids which equilibrate the oxygenated blood from the hepatic artery and the nutrient rich portal venous blood. Portal venous blood is less deoxygenated compared to the systemic veins.

Hepatocytes are polyhedral with central nucleus. Both the sides of the hepatocytes are exposed to the sinusoids. The cytoplasmic

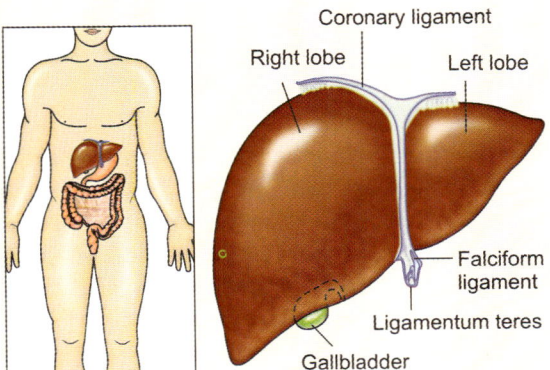

Fig. 1.1: Function of the liver

membrane of the hepatocytes has a specialized domain providing canalicular region on the lateral wall and numerous microvilli on the basolateral or sinusoidal surface.

The canalicular domains of the adjacent hepatocytes are bound together by tight junctions to form bile canaliculi.

Immunohistochemical techniques facilitate better identification of hepatocytes. Molecular techniques used for albumin or alpha fetoprotein synthesis also can identify the hepatocytes. Polyclonal carcinoembryonic antigen (CEA) stain bile canaliculi.

The functional unit of the liver is the acinus. Classically, the acinus is divided into three zones:

Zone 1 is around the portal tracts, is the most oxygenated and contains the highest concentration of nutrients and hormones.

Zone 3 is around the central vein and is poorly oxygenated.

Zone 2 is intermediate.

Each liver cell has two sinusoidal surfaces lined by microvilli. The sinusoidal surface is separated from the liver surface by the space of Disse. The canaliculi are formed by apposed liver cells and are also lined by microvilli. They are tight functional complexes between liver cells preventing bile leakage. The hepatocyte has a rough and smooth endoplasmic reticulum, golgi complexes, mitochondria, lysosome, peroxisomes, glycogen, and fat.

Sinusoids

The human sinusoids vary from 223 to 477 µm in length and 6 to 30 µm in diameter and can increase to 180 µm when necessary. Compared to sinusoidal diameter, the leukocytes are large so that blood flow compresses the sinusoidal wall, promoting exchange between plasma, subendothelial fluid and hepatocytes.

There are three types of sinusoidal cells:

Endothelial cells: They line the sinusoids in a discontinuous pattern. There are openings within endothelial cells called fenestrae which permit free movement between sinusoidal lumen and space of Disse.

Kupffer cells: They are located between the endothelial cells or on their surface. They have a macrophage like function and contain cytokines like tumor necrosis factor, interleukins, interferon.

Stellate cells: They store vitamin A and secrete extracellular collagens. They are type I collagen in the space of Disse.

The secretions of the liver are drained by right and left bile ducts which join together to form a common hepatic duct. This is soon joined by a cystic duct from the gallbladder to form the common bile duct. It runs anterior to the portal vein and to the right of the hepatic artery. It passes behind the first part of the duodenum in a groove on the back of the head of the pancreas usually joining by the main pancreatic duct to form the ampulla of Vater. The ampulla makes the duodenal mucosa to bulge inwards to form an eminence known as duodenal papilla where this duct opens in the second part of duodenum. In about 10–15% of subjects the two ducts, *viz.* common bile duct and pancreatic duct open separately into the duodenum.

Lymphatic Drainage The lymphatic vessel terminate in small groups of lymph nodes around the porta hepatis. The efferent vessels drain into glands around the celiac axis. Some superficial lymphatic vessels pass through the diaphragm to reach the mediastinal lymph nodes . Another small group drains into small lymph nodes around the intrathoracic portion of the inferior vena cava.

Thus porta hepatis has hepatic artery, portal vein, and the common bile duct.

The inferior vena cava is posterior to the liver, makes a deep groove to the right of the caudate lobe, about 2 cm from the midline.

The gallbladder lies in the fossa on the inferior surface of the right lobe.

The liver and related structures are richly supplied by sympathetic and parasympathetic nerve supply.

The liver is covered by the peritoneum and is kept in position by peritoneal ligaments and intra-abdominal pressure transmitted by the tone of the abdominal muscles.

The liver architecture is built on a reticulin framework which acts like a scaffolding. The basic architecture is in the form of hepatic lobules. The lobules are separated by thin septae. Each lobule has at the center a radical of the central hepatic vein. At the periphery is a portal triad containing branches of the hepatic artery, portal vein, and bile duct. The columns of the liver cells radiate from the central vein to the periphery interlaced in an orderly fashion by sinusoids.

Functions of the Liver

1. *Storage* Glycogen, vitamins (A, D, E, K and B12), and minerals
2. *Synthesis* Several vital proteins, e.g. albumin, prothrombin, fibrinogen
3. *Drug metabolism*
4. *Detoxification*
5. *Role in immune system* Through Kupffer's cells. It is a type of fixed macrophage which clears bacteria, fungi, parasites, worn out blood cells and cellular debris.

B. BILIRUBIN METABOLISM

Bilirubin is the final end product of the metabolism of the heme and other heme containing proteins such as cytochrome P450, myoglobin, and immature cells of the bone marrow. About 300 mg of bilirubin is formed daily of which 80–85% is derived from the haem and a small fraction from haem-proteins.

Haemoglobin is haem + globin. Haem is an iron-pigment. When senescent RBCs are lysed, the haemoglobin is broken into globin and haem moiety. Haem consists of a tetrapyrrole ring at the centre of which is an iron molecule.

When haem is broken by microsomal haem oxygenase (Fig. 1.2).

1. An iron atom is released which is re-utilized,
2. CO is excreted via lungs,

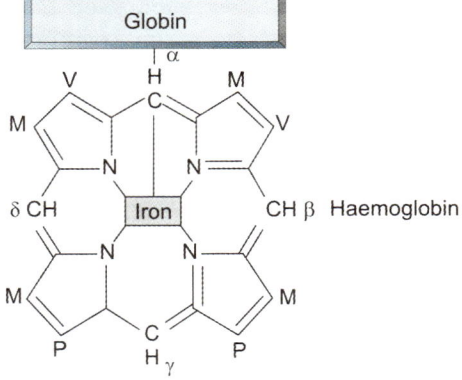

Fig. 1.2: Heam

3. The remaining green tetrapyrrolic moiety is called as biliverdin,
4. Biliverdin is subsequently reduced by biliverdin reductase to bilirubin. Bilirubin production averages about 4 mg/kg/day in a normal human being.

Since bilirubin is a potentially toxic waste product, the liver eliminates it from the body via the biliary tract.

The bilirubin after haem degradation is unconjugated and is poorly soluble. It is bound to a high affinity site on the plasma albumin and this unconjugated bilirubin-albumin complex is brought to the hepatocytes. The transfer of bilirubin to the bile involves:

1. Hepatocellular bilirubin uptake by dissociation from albumin.
2. Binding to specific intracellular cytosolic proteins.
3. Conjugation with glucuronic acid, catalyzed by diphospho-glucuronosyl transferase.
4. Canalicular excretion of conjugated bilirubin which is water-soluble.

Conjugated bilirubin which is excreted in the bile passes through the small intestine without significant absorption. It reaches the colon where it is deconjugated probably by bacterial β gluronidase, further degraded by bacterial enzymes to urobilinogen and other products. Urobilinogen is excreted in the stools as stercobilnogen (Fig. 1.3).

Some urobilinogen is reabsorbed from the colon which is **re-excreted** by the liver (enterohepatic circulation) but a small fraction is eliminated by the kidney.

Hyperbilirubinaemia may result from various causes: A acquired B congenital or familial.

A. Acquired

1. Excessive hemolysis (Pre-hepatic)
2. Liver disease (Hepatic)
3. Biliary obstruction (Post-hepatic)

B. The familial hyperbilirubinaemias can be classified into two categories:

I. Unconjugated hyperbilirubinaemia

1. Due to increased bilirubin production, e.g. congenital haemolytic anaemia, and
2. Shunt hyperbilirubinaemia.
   a. Congenital dyserythropoietic syndrome
   b. Miscellaneous

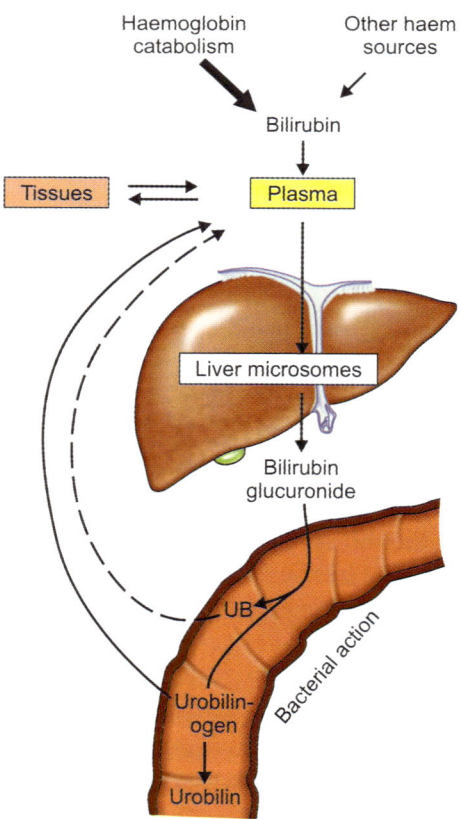

Fig. 1.3: Bilirubin metabolism

Defective Hepatic Clearance

Gilbert syndrome

Crigler-Najjar syndrome

a. Type I: phenobarbitone resistant
b. Type II: phenobarbitone responsive

II. Conjugated hyperbilirubinaemia

a. Dubin-Johnson syndrome
b. Rotor syndrome.

C. JAUNDICE

Jaundice is defined as yellowish discoloration of the sclera, mucous membrane and skin due to deposition of bilirubin in the elastic tissue of these structures because of circulating hyperbilirubinaemia. Hyperkeratonemia and mepacrine therapy may result into yellowness of the skin therefore, yellow discoloration of the sclera is more reliable sign of jaundice. A beginner may also differentiate it from muddy sclera as seen in Indian patients.

Icterus derived from a Greek word **ikteros** meaning *yellow* colour is also used synonymously with jaundice.

Jaundice may be noticed by:

a. **Examination of the sclera:** A patient is asked to look down towards his feet, the upper eyelid is lifted up so as to expose a larger area of the sclera and yellowness is noticed. It should be examined in a day light and not in artificial light.
b. Examination of the oral mucous membrane particularly over the hard palate.
c. Examination of the skin which shows yellowness in severe hyperbilirubinaemia.

Clinically the jaundice can be classified into the following types (Fig. 1.4):

1. Pre-hepatic: Increased production
2. Hepatic: Decreased clearance
3. Post-hepatic: Decreased excretion

Pre-hepatic: It is due to increased production of bilirubin due to excessive haemolysis or increased ineffective erythropoiesis.

Hepatic: The bilirubin production is within normal limits however due to diseased liver the bilirubin clearance is decreased ; resulting into hyperbilirubinaemia.

Post-hepatic: Since bilirubin is a potentially toxic waste product it is disposed by the liver, excreting it in the intestine via biliary tract. Pathology such as obstruction in the biliary tract results into accumulation of bilirubin in the blood.

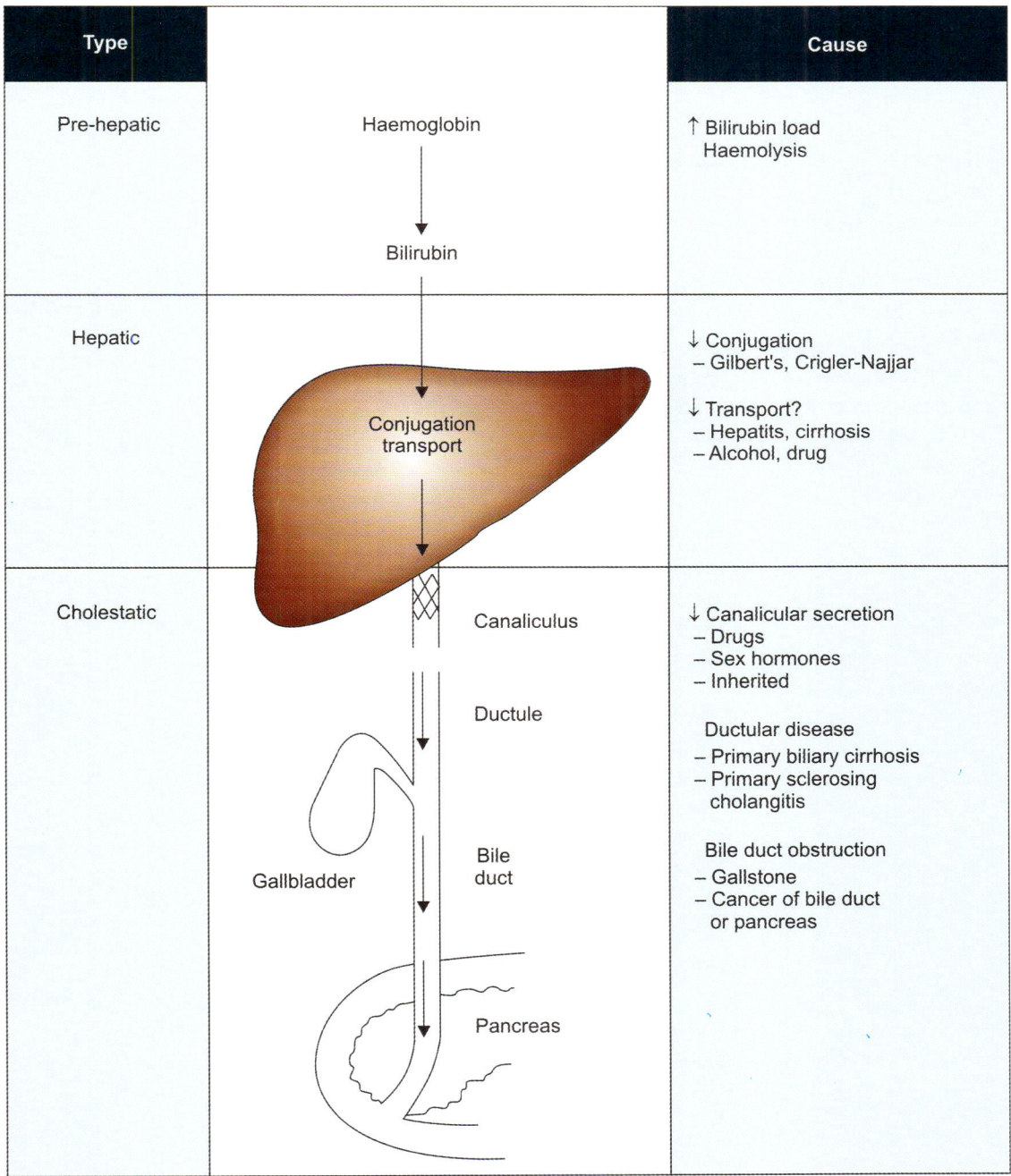

Type		Cause
Pre-hepatic	Haemoglobin ↓ Bilirubin	↑ Bilirubin load Haemolysis
Hepatic	Conjugation transport	↓ Conjugation – Gilbert's, Crigler-Najjar ↓ Transport? – Hepatits, cirrhosis – Alcohol, drug
Cholestatic	Canaliculus Ductule Gallbladder Bile duct Pancreas	↓ Canalicular secretion – Drugs – Sex hormones – Inherited Ductular disease – Primary biliary cirrhosis – Primary sclerosing cholangitis Bile duct obstruction – Gallstone – Cancer of bile duct or pancreas

Fig. 1.4: Classification of Jaundice

Jaundice is not a diagnosis. It is both a symptom and a sign.

The clinical approach to a case of jaundice.

1. *Colour of the sclera:* Yellowish discoloration of the sclera is jaundice. A lemon yellow colour (mild jaundice) suggests pre-hepatic jaundice as the bilirubin clearance by the liver is normal. Therefore, only a small increase is seen in unconjugated bilirubin in the blood. Hepatic jaundice is deep yellow in colour while post-hepatic or obstructive jaundice is very deep with an orange-green hue.

2. Scratch marks due to excessive itching are seen in post-hepatic jaundice. Patient complains of severe itching.

3. Clay coloured stools (chalky white) are seen in obstructive jaundice as stercobilinogen does not reach the intestine.

4. If a distended gallbladder is palpable at the tip of the right 9th costal cartilage it is more often due to malignant obstruction than a benign lesion.

Pre-hepatic jaundice: It is due to increased production of bilirubin, due to excessive breakdown of RBCs, i.e. haemolysis as in cases of distinct haemolytic disorders like inherited haemoglobinopathies, enzyme deficiencies, abnormalities of RBC cell membrane as well as acquired haemolytic anaemias.

In inherited haemolytic disorders, patient is anaemic, there may be a history of recurrent episodes of mild jaundice. Other siblings also may be affected. Since the RBCs are haemolyzed in the spleen, splenomegaly is present. Indirect bilirubin is raised, liver enzyme levels are normal.

Hepatic jaundice: It is due to disease of the liver and classified into the following:

a. Inflammatory: Hepatitis
b. Degenerative: Cirrhosis
c. Hepatotoxic drugs
d. Malignant neoplasms

Depending on the severity of the liver injury, the amount and type of circulating bilirubin will vary. Both indirect and direct bilirubin levels are raised. In addition, the liver enzymes are increased due to hepatic injury.

Post-hepatic jaundice: It is due to obstructive lesions like stones, strictures, malignancies obstructing biliary excretion. Jaundice is deep, direct or conjugated hyperbilirubinaemia is seen. Serum alkaline phosphatase is raised. Patients complains of clay coloured stools and itching.

D. SIGNS OF HEPATIC DYSFUNCTION OR LIVER CELL FAILURE

The chronic liver cell injury results into fibrosis and degeneration of the hepatocytes. Whenever degeneration exceeds the regenerative capacity of the liver it clinically manifests with signs of liver cell failure. Cirrhosis is taken as a prototype of chronic liver cell injury and signs of hepatic dysfunction are discussed here.

Signs of Liver Cell Failure

1. Chronic ill-health
2. Fever and Gram-negative septicaemia
3. Skin changes
4. Endocrine changes
5. Haematological disorders
6. Hyperdynamic circulation
7. Jaundice
8. Ascites
9. Hepatic pre-encephalopathy
10. Hepatic encephalopathy
11. Fetor hepaticus.

Ascites and hepatic encephalopathy are discussed in subsequent chapters.

Chronic Ill-Health

Patient complains of fatigability and weakness. He may develop wasting of the muscles due to difficulty in synthesising tissue proteins, malnutrition, etc.

Fever and Gram-negative Septicemia

Cirrhotic patient may get continuously low grade fever which can be explained on the basis of certain cytokines particularly tumour necrosis factor.

In addition, bacteria from intestinal flora may enter the systemic circulation by passing through porto-systemic collaterals or they get an entry to the systemic circulation through defective hepatic filter.

Grade C cirrhotics are usually affected and recurrent episodes are bad prognostic factors. The hospital mortality is about 38%. Ominous features are absence of fever, marked leucocytosis, and elevated serum creatinine.

Skin Changes

1. *Spider naevi:* They consist of a central arteriole from which small vessels radiate resembling spider's legs (Fig 1.5 a and b). If the central arteriole is pressed with pin's head, the radiating vessels blanch. The spider naevi are usually seen above the nipple line.
2. *Paper money skin:* Like vascular spider, many small vessels may be randomly scattered through the skin like silk thread in currency notes. It is known as paper money skin.
3. *Palmer erythema:* Palms are warm and bright red in colour especially thenar and hypo-thenar eminences and finger pulps. It is particularly seen in decompensated cirrhosis. It is due to vasodilatation and hyperdynamic circulation. Palmer flushing and bounding pulses are common. It may be difficult to appreciate it in coloured people.
4. *Chalky white nails:* The nails are chalky white with a pink zone at the tip of the nail. Whiteness is due to opacity of the nail bed.

The aetiology of the skin changes mostly remains unknown. It is postulated that high levels of circulating oestrogen cause vascular changes (also seen in pregnancy) and are the cause of spider naevi and palmer erythema.

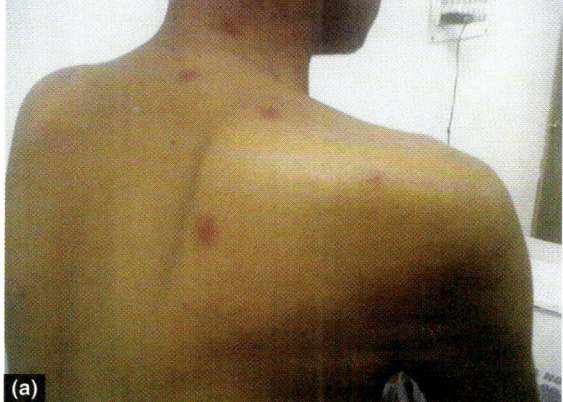
(a)

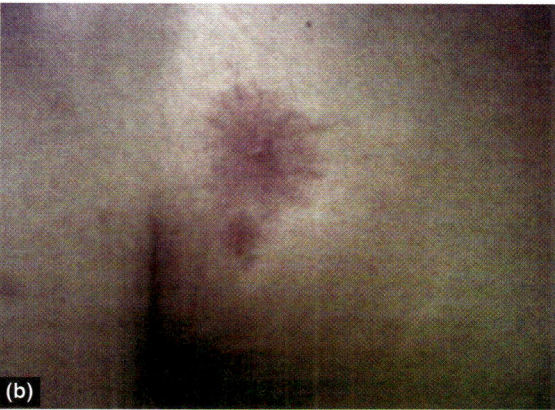
(b)

Fig. 1.5 a and b: Spider naevi

Oestrogen is inactivated by normal liver but it is seen that in cirrhosis, oestradiol/free testosterone ratio is high in males having spiders.

Endocrine Changes

Endocrine changes are mainly related to sex hormones or gonadal failure. Libido and potency is diminished. Infertility is common.

The secondary sex characters are affected. Loss of axillary and pubic hair (not the scalp hair with which one in born) is seen.

In males, decreased frequency of shaving suggests reduced beard and mustache.

Feminisation is noted in males. There is gynaecomastia [enlargement of the breast (Fig. 1.6)]. Testicular atrophy is common. The testes are smaller in size and soft.

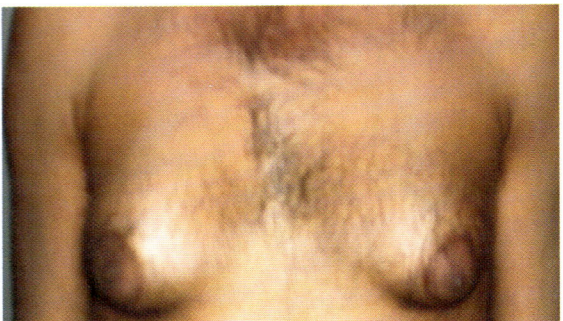

Fig. 1.6: Gynaecomastia

Normal testes are firm, testicular sensation is preserved.

Females with cirrhosis lose feminine characteristics notably loss of breast and pelvic fat. Pubic and axillary hair are sparse. Menstrual irregularities and infertility is common.

Mechanism. The sources of oestrogens (oestrogen, oestradiol, oestriol) in men are adrenals, testes and peripheral conversion of major circulating androgens.

Human liver has receptors both for oestrogens and andogens.In cirrhosis,the hepatic androgen receptors fall and hepatic oestrogen receptor concentration increases. It results in increased sensitivity to oestrogens.

Secondly, the metabolism of hormones by the liver may be decreased due to decrease in hepatic blood flow seen in cirrhotics.

Cirrhotics with ascites may also show secondary hyperaldosteronism as well as increase ADH levels.

Hematological Disorders

Increased red cell destruction is invariably seen in hepatocellular failure. The hepatocytes synthesize all coagulation factors except von Willebrand's and factor VIII C.

The liver synthesizes vitamin K dependent factors II,VII, IX, X as well as labile factor V. Plasma prothrombin is low and falls with fall in serum protein levels.

All these deficiencies may cause bleeding diathesis in terminally ill-patients. Splenomegaly due to portal hypertension may be responsible for anaemia, leucopaenia, thrombocytopaenia due to hypersplenism.

Changes in nitrogen metabolism. Serum albumin levels go on decreasing as the severity of the cirrhosis increases. There is a reversal of serum albumin/globulin ratio.

As the liver functions deteriorate, liver is unable to convert ammonia to urea as a result serum ammonia levels increase.

Urea production is also impaired.

Fetor hepaticus. Severe hepatocellular disease with extensive collateral circulation produces fetor hepaticus, i.e. a faecal smell of the breath. It is similar to freshly opened corpse or mice.

Patients with fetor hepaticus have increased levels of methyl mercaptan in urine. It is probably of intestinal origin. This substance is exhaled in the breath giving the characteristic fetor. It is probably derived from methionine. The de-methylating processes are inhibited in the presence of the liver damage.

Investigations in a Case of Cirrhosis

1. **Liver function tests:** In a decompensated cirrhosis, the liver functions are deranged.

   In absence of acute cellular injury, liver enzymes are not markedly elevated but the rise in SGOT and SGPT is mild to moderate. Serum bilirubin may be increased. The reversal of albumin/globulin ratio is characteristically seen in these patients.

   Prothrombin time is prolonged.

2. **Ultrasonography:** It is not reliable for diagnosis of cirrhosis but is good to screen for hepatic malignancy.

   Ultrasonography shows:

   1. The size of the liver which may be shrunken in advanced disease.
   2. Liver echotexture is heterogenous depending on the severity of the fibrosis. In advanced condition it is coarse.
   3. It shows portal vein which is dilated in cases of portal hypertension. Portal collaterals may be seen. It evaluates

portal vein patency. The Doppler study is done for direction of portal blood flow.

4. Presence of ascites is detected by USG.
5. Hepatocellular carcinoma in cirrhosis due to HBV and HCV can be seen.
6. Splenomegaly is noticed.

CT scan. It can assess the size, shape, and nodularity of the liver. Fatty changes and space occupying lesions can be recognized. Contrast study evaluates portal circulation and collaterals. Splenomegaly confirms portal hypertension. Ascites is seen.
- CT gives an objective evaluation.
- CT guided biopsy can be performed safely.

Liver Biopsy

Liver biopsy is the gold standard of diagnosing cirrhosis of the liver. It shows the characteristic parenchymal changes. It is diagnostic of cirrhosis. It shows degenerative changes in the form of hepatocyte degeneration, fibrous septae, absence of portal triads, and regenerating nodules. Abnormal vascular arrangement is noted. It also contributes to the aetiology of the cirrhosis. The limitation of the test are:

1. It is invasive.
2. Rarely it may cause bleeding in the liver.
3. A tiny piece is available for examination. It is not possible to quantify the severity of fibrosis.
4. Expensive.
5. Variable subjective interpretations.

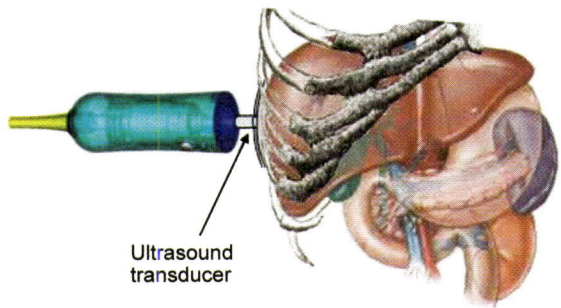

Ultrasound transducer

Fig. 1.7: Fibroscan

The other tests are:

1. Fibroscan
2. Other imaging techniques
3. Biochemical markers

1. **Fibroscan:** The Fibroscan device (echosens) works by measuring shear wave velocity. In this technique, a 50-MHz wave is passed into the liver from a small transducer on the end of an ultrasound probe (Fig. 1.7). The probe also has a transducer on the end that can measure the velocity of the shear wave (in metres per second) as this wave passes through the liver. The shear wave velocity can then be converted into liver stiffness, which is expressed in kilopascals. Essentially, the technology measures the velocity of the sound wave passing through the liver and then converts that measurement into a liver stiffness measurement; the entire process is often referred to as liver ultrasonographic elastography.

   It is a measure of liver fibrosis. The stiffness of the liver due to fibrosis can be assessed by non-invasive method. It can be performed by the bedside of the patient. It is reliable and reproducible. There is no risk of pain or bleeding. Compared to liver biopsy it is less expensive. The limitations are:
   1. Presence of ascites
   2. Morbid obesity
   3. Thick chest wall

2. **Other imaging techniques:** They are as follows:
   a. *MRI elastography:* One radiologic method for measuring liver fibrosis is magnetic resonance (MR) elastography. The advantage of MR elastography is that it is very accurate for measuring liver stiffness; however, this test requires patients to undergo an MR imaging scan, and therefore it cannot be performed at the point of care. It is expensive.
   b. *Acoustic resonance force impulse testing:* It is another radiologic method for measuring liver fibrosis, but this method is still undergoing evaluation.

3. Several non-invasive tests use **serum biomarkers** to determine liver fibrosis. These tests make use of the fact that changes in liver stiffness lead to measurable changes in the biomarkers produced by the liver. Serum biomarker tests measure one or more of these biomarkers and look for elevated levels of those biomarkers that are associated with fibrosis. The most common serum tests for staging liver fibrosis are: HepaScore, FibroSure, the FIB-4 index, and the European liver fibrosis test.

General Management of these Conditions

Liver architecture which is damaged in cirrhosis never regains normal structure. However, regenerative capacity of the normal hepatocytes is enormous which can restore functional compensation though structural changes do not return to normal. When degeneration is more than regeneration, clinically the signs of liver cell failure are seen.

The liver cell dysfunctions are precipitated by GI bleed, alcoholic episodes, acute infections, electrolyte disturbances due to diarrhoea—vomiting or induced by diuretics, abdominal paracentesis. These conditions need prompt medical management.

Bedrest. It reduces functional demands on the liver. It is continued if functional improvement is noted. But if condition does not improve after 4 weeks of rest, moderate activity is permitted.

Diet. In absence of encephalopathy, a high caloric (2500 cal/day) diet containing 80–100 gm of proteins is advocated; particularly in alcoholics. Deficiencies of folic acid, vitamin B complex, trace elements need to be attended to.

Alcohol. patient must abstain from alcohol.
- *Anaemia:* Haemoglobin level should be kept above 10 gm/100 ml.
- *Hormone therapy:* Steroids, sex hormones including oral testosterone have no role.

- *Sedatives:* May be used sparingly. Morphine is likely to precipitate coma, must be avoided.
- *Barbiturates:* Long acting, short-chain barbiturates like phenobarbitone are excreted by kidneys, small doses are tolerated by cirrhotics.
- Chlordizepoxide causes oversedation and should be avoided.
- Oxazepam may remain the drug of choice.
- Management of encephalopathy and other signs of failure are discussed in subsequent chapters.

E. ASCITES (GENERAL CONSIDERATION)

Ascites is a pathological collection of fluid in the peritoneal cavity.

The word ascites is derived from Greek language (*askos* refers to *a bag* or *a sac*). This word is a noun used singularly. The adjective is ascitic as in ascitic fluid (and not ascites fluid).

Due to gravity initially the fluid in the peritoneal cavity gets collected in the pelvis. As the amount of fluid increases it collects in the abdominal recesses as in paracolic gutters. The flanks are bulging, gradually abdominal distension goes on increasing, the umbilicus is either transversely stretched (smiling umbilicus) or is everted. Distension of abdomen is clinically apparent. If massive, it may cause respiratory embarrassment. Patient complains of breathlessness particularly on lying down.

As the ascites goes on increasing the intravascular circulating volume decreases as a result of which the patient develops oliguria. It may also be accompanied by the oedema feet.

Examination of the Abdomen

Inspection : Fullness in flanks is seen.
: Abdominal distension is noticed.
: Veins of the abdominal wall may be visible due to stretching of the abdominal wall.

: Umbilicus is transversely stretched or everted.

: If ascites of a longer duration, divarication of rectii is noted. Patient in supine position is asked to raise his head, divarication is seen as a gap between the two rectii muscles.

Palpation : Abdomen is superficially palpated for any lumps, a doughy feeling, tenderness, etc. Ascites due to tuberculosis feels doughy on palpation.

In presence of massive ascites, dipping method is used to detect organomegaly, *viz.* hepato-splenomegaly. The anterior abdominal wall is pressed by pressure of both hands displacing the fluid so as to palpate the deeper organs. If ascites is moderate to massive, the fluid thrill can be elicited. The examiner keeps his palm on one side of the abdomen and taps the abdominal wall on the opposite side. These vibrations are conducted through the fluid and felt by palm on the opposite side as a thrill. To dampen the vibrations conducted through the abdominal wall a patient is asked to place his hand in the midline on the abdominal wall.

Percussion

Minimal fluid in the pelvis is detected by sonography as presence of fluid in the pouch of Douglas.

Minimal fluid in the abdomen is detected by Puddle's sign. Patient is in knee-elbow position. In this position fluid if any gravitates around umbilicus. Percussion around umbilicus gives dull note due to presence of fluid.

Moderate ascites is detected by 'horseshoe' dullness. It is due to accumulation of fluid in the paracolic recesses. One starts percussion in the midline from xiphisternum downwards. In ascites a dull note is heard at some point. From this point percussion is continued radially till the dull note is heard. When all these dull points are joined it gives a shape of a horseshoe with open end facing xiphisternum.

The abdomen is percussed from xiphisternum downwards in the midline till one gets a dull note indicating presence of fluid. From this point the abdomen is percussed laterally to the flank, till a point of maximum dullness is reached, without changing the pleximetre finger, patient is asked to turn/rotate on the other side. The same point is percussed again. The earlier dull note is replaced by a tympanic note as the free fluid shifts to the other flank to the dependent part and intestines floating over the fluid impart tympanic note.

Shifting dullness is a very important sign. Shifting dullness indicates **free fluid** (fluid is free to shift from one flank to the other. It is not seen in encysted fluid collection, e.g. large ovarian cyst).

In a massive ascites it may be difficult to elicit shifting dullness as there is no space for the fluid to shift. Fluid thrill can be elicited.

Auscultation. Abdomen is ascultated for peristaltic sounds.

In addition one may look for venus hum, arterial bruit, etc.

Causes of Ascites

- Cirrhosis of liver
- Tubercular peritonitis
- Malignant ascites
- Ascites as a part of generalized anasarca
  – Anaemia-hypoproteinaemia
  – Nephrotic syndrome
  – Congestive heart failure
- IVC obstruction
- Budd-Chiari syndrome: veno-occlusive disease.

Once clinically concluded that it is a case of ascites one has to answer the following questions:

Q.1. Where is the lesion?
Ans. Peritoneal cavity.

Q.2. What is the lesion?
Ans. Pathological accumulation of fluid.

Q.3. What is the aetiology of the lesion?

Ans. When a patient presents with ascites one should first consider ascites due to cirrhosis of the liver.

Infective. Mostly due to tuberculous peritonitis.

Malignancy. Malignant spread to the peritonium.

Clinical examination, relevant investigations based on clinical diagnosis, diagnostic tapping of the ascitic fluid will help to arrive at a diagnosis.

Salient features of these conditions are discussed below for bedside diagnosis.

Cirrhosis of the Liver

Ascites is a sign of a decompensated cirrhosis as such it is present in an advanced stage of cirrhosis. Therefore, other stigmatas of cirrhosis may be present and should be carefully examined, e.g. spider naevi, palmer erythema, gynaecomastia, jaundice, etc.

In cirrhosis, ascites is due to hypoalbuminaemia. Portal hypertension limits the fluid collection to the peritoneal cavity. In cirrhosis the ascites is followed by the oedema feet which is usually mild to moderate.

Oedema feet is due to hypoproteinaemia. It is further contributed by functional block of inferior vena cava due to pressure of the abdominal fluid.

Long-standing ascites with increased intra-abdominal pressure favours diastasis rectii (divarication), and may result into umbilical hernia which is seen in about 20% of cases. Femoral and inginal hernias also may be present. The risk is of rupture or incarceration.

In a tense ascites, it is difficult to detect hepatosplenomegaly. Although spleen is difficult to palpate it does not rule out portal hypertension.

The very fact that ascites is disproportionately much more than oedema feet, indicates the presence of the portal hypertension which limits the collection of fluid to the peritoneal

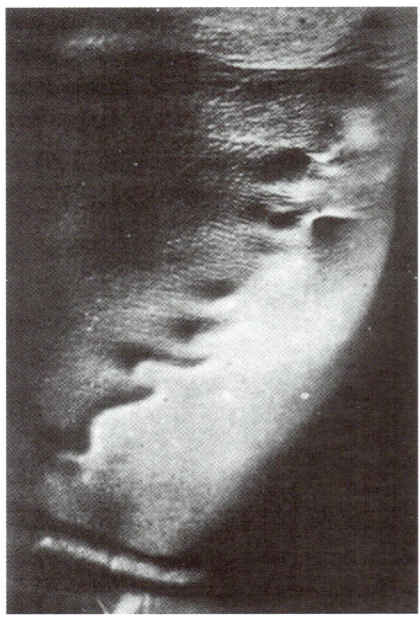

Fig. 1.8: An anterior abdominal wall vein in a patient with cirrhosis of the liver

cavity. In fact, it is portal hypertension which initiates the fluid leak in the peritoneal cavity.

Therefore, sign of portal hypertension should be looked for. Dilated tortuous veins may be noticed on the abdominal wall (Fig. 1.8). Veins radiating from the umbilicus may be noticed as caput medusae. A venous hum may be heard in the epigastric region.

Cruveilhier-Baumgarten syndrome. A venous hum is heard in the epigastrium or near the umbilicus over a congenitally patent umbilical vein. Portal hypertension opens up portosystemic collaterals. One of the sites is veins of the abdominal wall. Increased flow across the umbilical vein causes a venous hum.

Relevant investigations include liver function tests, abdominal sonography, ascitic paracentesis for cytochemistry and liver biopsy. Ascitic fluid is transudate.

Ascites due to peritoneal tuberculosis. A patient presents with symptoms of tuberculosis like low-grade fever, loss of appetite, weight loss and gradually increasing ascites.

The stigmata of cirrhosis are absent. The abdomen may feel doughy. Signs of ascites are present.

Ultrasonography (USG) of abdomen shows fluid in the abdomen which may show presence of fibrous strands. Abdominal lymphadenopathy may be noted. Peritoneoscopy may reveal peritoneal tubercles.

Ascitic fluid is straw coloured, may at times be haemorrhagic. Being infective/inflammatory fluid the protein content is high, cell count is raised with predominant lymphocytosis (exudate).

TB PCR of the ascitic fluid or TB culture gives microbiological diagnosis.

Malignant ascites. Symptoms and signs of primary tumour may be present. In about 20% cases the primary malignancy may remain undetected. History suggestive of malignancy, Imaging techniques and tumour markers may help to detect the primary malignancy. Paracentesis of ascitic fluid is haemorrhagic with high content of proteins and presence of malignant cells.

Ascites as a Part of Generalised Anasarca (Differential Diagnosis)

Anaemia-hypoproteinaemia. The patient is severely pale. Cutaneous signs of hypoproteinaemia may be present. Fluid overload manifests first with puffiness of the face, followed by oedema feet and then generalised anasarca of which ascites is a part. Haemic murmur may be present. Usually, the cause is nutritional. Complete blood count (CBC) and serum protein estimation helps the diagnosis. Red cell indices and serum iron studies confirms the deficiency anaemia. Ascitic fluid is transudate. Cause of anaemia needs to be treated. Hematinics and protein suppliments correct the condition.

Nephrotic syndrome. Syndrome is characterized by proteinuria, hypoalbuminaemia, anasarca and hyper-cholesterolaemia. Patient presents with puffiness of face, oliguria, oedema feet and ascites as a part of generalized anasarca. Urinary proteins, serum albumin and cholesterol estimations are carried out to confirm the syndrome. Further investigations are carried out to ascertain the cause of the nephrotic syndrome. Renal biopsy may be necessary for diagnosis. Treatment of the cause, protein suppliments and steroids as and when indicated are the mainstay of the treatment.

Congestive heart failure (CHF). Clinical profile is related to basic cardiac lesion either congenital or acquired. Three cardinal signs of CHF are 1 raised JVP 2 oedema feet 3 congestive hepatomegaly. Ascites is a part of fluid overload.

Inferior vena caval (IVC) obstruction. Patient presents with oedema feet, dilated veins on the lower abdominal wall with reversal of blood flow from below upwards.

Budd-Chiari syndrome—Veno-occlusive disease. The venous occlusion may be at various levels; from the efferent veins from the acinus, intra and extrahepatic course of the hepatic veins, enty of hepatic vein into IVC, and finally IVC opening in the right atrium.

The most common cause of thrombosis of the hepatic veins is due to conditions causing thrombophilia such as deficiency of protein S, protein C, myeloproliferative disorder, polycythaemia and local compression by the tumours. The incidence is about 1 in 100, 000. Clinical features vary from asymptomatic patient to acute liver failure. Usually, patient complains of right upper quadrant pain, hepatomegaly, and ascites. Jaundice and splenomegaly are usually mild.

Similar clinical picture is mimicked by constrictive pericarditis.

2

Cirrhosis of the Liver

Alaka Deshpande

CIRRHOSIS OF THE LIVER

Cirrohosis of the liver depicts a specific histopathological picture. However, with a constellation of symptoms and signs, a fairly accurate clinical diagnosis of cirrhosis can be made.

Cirrhosis is derived from the Greek word **kirrhos** meaning *yellow-orange*.

In 1761, Gianbattisla Morgagni published a report of 500 autopsies and first time identified a peculiar transformation of the liver. However, the name cirrhosis, meaning *yellowish tan colour*, was given by Laennec in 1826. The parenchymal degeneration, regeneration and scarring was reported by Roselle as pathogenesis.

WHO classification of cirrhosis:

- Morphological
  - Macronodular
  - Micronodular
  - Mixed
- Histological
- Portal
- Infective
- Biliary
- Congestive
- Aetiologic
- Genetic, infective, toxic, biliary, vascular, cryptogenic.

Cirrohosis can be defined as a degenerative process resulting from a chronic liver injury causing collapse of the reticulin framework of the liver with extensive fibrosis (wound healing process) and regeneration of hepatocytes resulting into nodular transformation.

It is important to remember:

1. There are variety of causes incriminated for chronic liver injury (Fig. 2.1).
2. A degenerative process implies the ongoing process with irreversibility.

However, with better understanding of the injury and the therapeutic advances have shown that removal of underlying insult can reverse the fibrosis, e.g.

1. Treatment of hepatitis B virus (HBV), hepatitis C virus (HCV) infections
2. Treatment of haemochromatosis
3. Cessation of alcohol intake.

Only nodular transformation without fibrosis is not cirrhosis.

Only fibrosis is not synonymous with cirrhosis.

A fibrous reaction due to ova is seen in schistosomiasis but it does not evolve into cirrhosis.

Degeneration due to chronic liver injury which is healing by fibrosis and a regeneration of normal hepatocytes is going on simultaneously. For a longtime therefore the liver functions remain within normal limits, clinically the patient remains asymptomatic. This stage of the disease is called as a compensated cirrhosis of the liver.

But whenever hepatic functions are compromised due to degeneration being more than regeneration, patient develops symptoms of liver cell failure/hepatic dysfunction, it is called as a decompensated cirrhosis of the liver.

The clinical presentation of the cirrhosis may be due to:

1. Hepatic dysfunction *per se* as well as
2. Sequelae of cirrhosis like portal hypertension.

PATHOGENESIS OF CIRRHOSIS

Liver cirrhosis is the final pathological result of various chronic liver injuries/diseases. There is a large variation in the aetiologies of cirrhosis but the pathological characteristics are mostly common for all the cirrhotic cases including degeneration and necrosis of hepatocytes, replacement of hepatic parenchyma by fibrosis and regenerative nodules which finally decompensate and result into loss of liver function. Fibrosis is the precursor of cirrhosis and plays a pivotal role in pathogenesis.

The liver architecture is built on a reticulin framework which acts like a scaffolding. It comprises of a group of macromolecules also referred to as extracellular matrix (ECM). The macro-molecules include collagen, non-collagen glycoproteins, matrix bound growth factors, proteoglycans, and matricellular proteins.

Following liver injury/insults, various inflammatory cytokines such as platelet derived growth factor PDGF, transformin growth factor TGF beta, tumour necrosis factor TNF alpha, IL-1, activate the resting stellate cells (HSC). Activation of HSC is characterized by cell proliferation and migration, transformation into myofibroblasts, generation of a large amount of collagen and other ECM molecules ultimately resulting into liver fibrosis.

After the hepatic injury, there is a 3 to 8-fold increase in ECM. There is a loss of endothelial cell fenestrations and hepatocyte microvilli associated with the capillarization of sinusoids. These changes interfere and impede the metabolic exchange between the sinusoidal pool of blood and hepatocytes. The sinusoidal collapse raises the portal venous pressure.

The role of hepatocytes is complicated in fibrosis. These cells are targets for the most of the hepatotoxic agents like viruses, alcohol, toxins, drugs, etc.

Chronic liver injuries promote:

1. Apoptosis of hepatocytes, and
2. Trigger the compensatory regeneration of liver cells.

Apoptosis is a common sequel to liver injury and contributes to inflammation, fibrogenesis, and development of cirrhosis.

Hepatocyte Regeneration

Liver has a great capacity to regenerate. Whenever there is a need for additional hepatocytes, the quiescent cells are stimulated by primers and cytokines so that the cells are in a primed state. The growth factors stimulate DNA synthesis and cellular replication.

Priming is necessary for hepatocytes to respond to the growth factors. If injury/toxic attack persists causing massive loss of hepatocytes then liver cells may be derived from progenitor/stem cells either within the liver or the bone marrow.

Causes of Cirrhosis

1. Chronic alcoholism
2. Viral cirrhosis, chronic HBV, HCV, hepatitis D virus (HDV) infection
3. Non-alcoholic steatohepatitis (NASH)
4. Primary biliary cirrhosis (PBC)
5. Primary sclerosing cholangitis
6. Autoimmune hepatitis
7. Cardiac cirrhosis
8. Metabolic
   Haemochromatosis: iron overload
   Wilson's disease: copper overload
9. α-1, antitrypsin deficiency

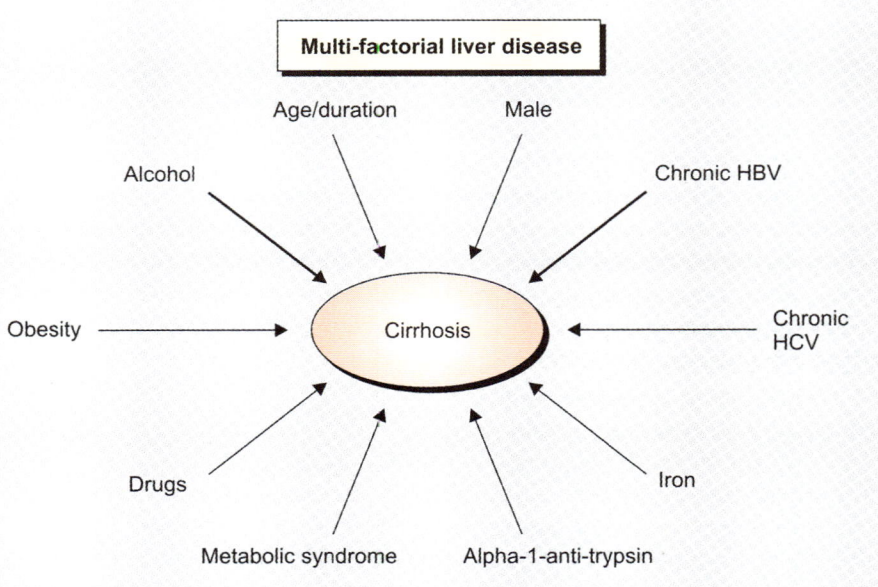

Fig. 2.1: Many liver diseases have a major initiating factor and a number of co-factors contributing to the development of cirrhosis.

10. Budd-Chiari syndrome
11. Toxins and drugs
    Methotrexate, amiodarone
12. Cryptogenic

Alcoholic Cirrhosis

Alcohol is the most frequently used and socially acceptable hepatotoxin worldwide. Alcohol affects the liver depending on the dose and duration of the use or abuse.

It is further compounded by post-alcohol nutritional intake, behavioural complexities under the effect of alcohol (multi-partner unprotected sex—a risk factor for acquisition of HBV, HIV infections, intra venous (IV) drug abuse a risk factor for HCV acquisition, etc.)

In developing countries like India the alcohol may be brewed differently, is adulterated and contains a lot of impurities and hepatotoxins.

Available evidence indicates increased risk of cirrhosis with ingestion of > 60–80 gm/day of alcohol in men and > 20 gm/day in women consumed for 10 years.

Histologic Manifestations of Alcoholic Liver Disease

These diseases are as follows:
- Fatty liver or steatosis
- Acute alcoholic hepatitis
- Chronic hepatitis
- Hepatic fibrosis
- Cirrhosis.

Alcohol Metabolism

Mainly three enzymes are involved in alcohol metabolism (Fig. 2.2).
1. Alcohol dehydrogenase
2. Acetaldehyde dehydrogenase
3. Cytochrome P450 system.

Alcohol is metabolized to acetaldehyde, which is extremely reactive and toxic.

Acetaldehyde has been shown to have the following hepatotoxic effects:
1. Induction of steatosis
2. Increasing sensitization to TNF α-mediated hepatocyte necrosis

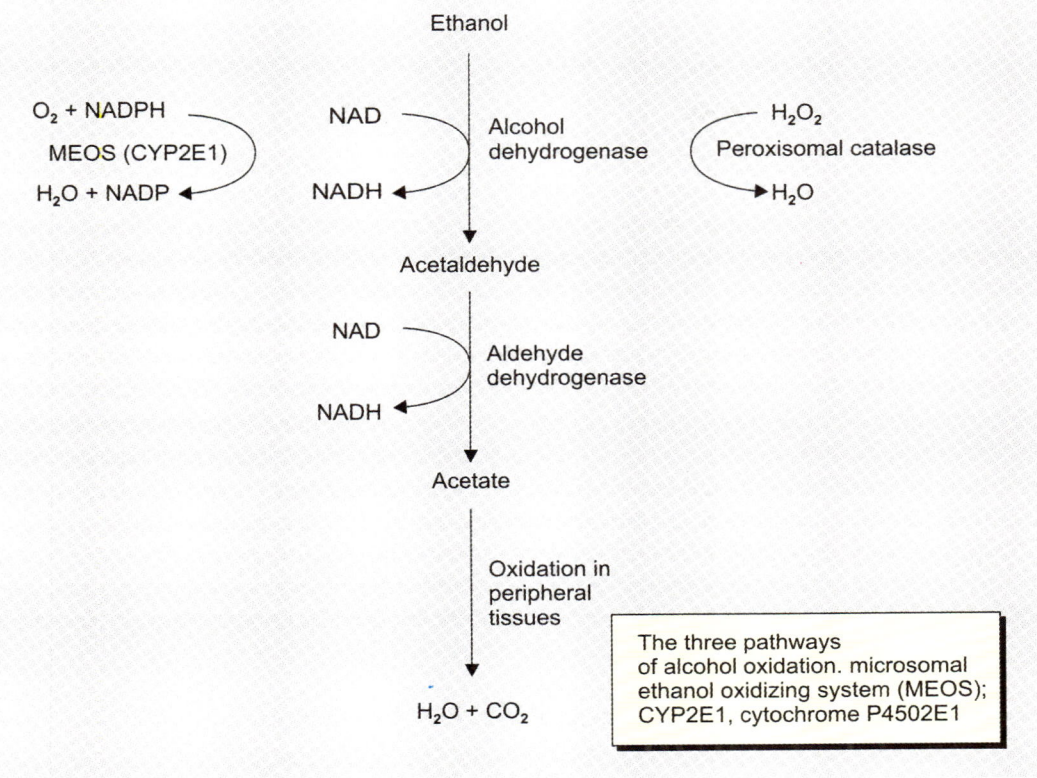

Fig. 2.2: Alcohol metabolism

3. Binding to host proteins.
   • Inducing endoplasmic reticular stress affecting the function, e.g. microtubules, and
   • Forming neo-antigens.

Oxidative stress. In alcoholic liver disease the generation of pro-oxidants overwhelms the endogeneous anti-oxidant systems. The pro-oxidants can directly come from ethanol metabolism or from activated phagocytes resulting into liver injury.

Clinically, various signs of liver cell failure as described earlier may be seen.

Other Features

The other features include bilateral parotid enlargement, loss of memory, insomnia, irritability, hallucinations, convulsions (rumfits), alcoholic tremors; all indicate alcohol dependence and should be distinguished from hepatic encephalopathy. Hepatorenal syndrome is common. Dupuytren's contractures of the palmer fascia are related to alcohol and not cirrhosis.

Gynaecomastia may appear after spironolactone therapy.

Alcoholic cardiomyopathy, hypertension, arrhythmias and coronary artery disease are also common.

Treatment

The most important measure is immediate abstinence from alcohol. It may cause withdrawal syndrome (delirium tremens) which should be treated. Other general measures remain the same.

Alcohol related liver disease accounts for 20–30% of all indications of liver transplant in the USA and UK.

CIRRHOSIS DUE TO HEPATITIS B, C, D

With the availability of diagnostic facilities in India, the number of hepatitis B and hepatitis C infected individuals is increasing. Hepatitis B is transmitted by sexual, parenteral and vertical (mother to child) routes.

Hepatitis C in transmitted parenterally and commonly seen in IV drug abusers. In India, currently all the blood units are being screened for hepatitis B and C. About 20% of cases exposed to HBV and HCV go on to develop cirrhosis after a period of 15 to 20 years.

Clinical features remain the same as in alcoholic cirrhosis.

Liver biopsy in HCV infection in addition to usual features of cirrhosis, shows inflammatory infiltrates in portal areas.

Management

It involves specific management of complications of cirrhosis. In addition, patient needs specific antiviral therapy as discussed in viral hepatitis. And finally liver transplant.

Non-alcoholic Fatty Liver Disease (NAFLD)

It is one of the most common liver disorders world over.

It is defined as liver fat more than 5–10% by weight and frequently taken as 5–10% macro-steatotic hepatocytes in biopsy specimen. The prevalence is closely associated with ethnicity and is influenced by familial factors. It is closely associated with:

- Obesity with insulin resistance
- Type 2 diabetes mellitus
- Metabolic syndrome
- Dyslipidemias
- Hepatic fat accumulation results from
  1. Uptake of circulating fatty acids from lipolysis of adipose tissue.
  2. Uptake of VLDL-derived low-density lipoprotein remnants.
  3. *De novo* lipogenesis from carbohydrate substrates.

Lipid peroxidation mediated by free radicals is the most common mechanism.

Nonalcoholic steatohepatitis (NASH), a type of non-alcoholic fatty liver disease (NAFLD) is characterized by inflammation, ballooned hepatocytes, cell death and fibrosis progressing to cirrhosis.

Autoimmune Hepatitis

The diagnosis is based on autoimmune markers like antinuclear antibodies (ANA), and antismooth muscle antibody (ASMA). Liver biopsy is not of much help. Many cases of autoimmune hepatitis present with cirrhosis and signs of active inflammation.

Immunosuppressive therapy will be beneficial.

Cardiac Cirrhosis

It is secondary to repeated episodes or long-term right-sided congestive cardiac failure. With increased awareness, improved diagnostics and early interventions the incidence of rheumatic valvular heart disease causing right sided heart failure has decreased now in India.

Right sided heart failure results into passive venous congestion of the liver causing hepatomegaly. Elevated venous pressure is transmitted to the liver sinusoids via hepatic veins. Due to reduced cardiac output, insult is further aggravated by hepatic ischaemia. Centrilobular hepatocytes can become necrotic leading to pericentral fibrosis. Portal hypertension is very very rare in such cases.

The treatment is based on management of underlying cardiac disease.

Iron Overload-Haemochromatosis

An increase in systemic iron levels is consequence of:

1. Hereditary haemochromatosis which results from mutation in HFE (high iron or ferrous) gene causing excessive intestinal absorption of dietary iron.
2. Ineffective erythropoiesis.
3. Parenteral iron administration.

Excessive intracellular deposition of iron damages tissues and organs. Symptomatic patients present with cirrhosis of liver, arthritis, dilated cardiomyopathy, skin pigmentation, diabetes secondary to pancreatitis, hypogonadism due to testicular atrophy and hypothyroidism. Elevated serum ferritin levels and transferrin saturation are diagnostic.

Hereditary haemochromatosis requires regular phlebotomies. Secondary haemochromatosis is managed with iron chelation.

Copper Overload—Wilson's Disease

It is an autosomal recessive disorder with specific mutations in ATP7B gene on chromosome 13.

There is a deficiency of circulating ceruloplasmin with defect in biliary excretion of the copper. As a result, the copper levels in the liver are high, more than 250 mg/gm dry weight of the liver. Copper also gets deposited in the basal gangalia. Presence of Kayser-Fleischer ring in the eye, stigmata of cirrhosis and signs of extrapyramidal lesion along with biochemical parameters helps in the diagnosis.

Copper chelation therapy is primary therapy in a symptomatic patient. Oral penicillamine 750–1000 mg/day in divided dosage is given. Efficacy is measured by urinary Cu > 250 µg/day, non-ceruloplasmin Cu < 10 µg.

Primary Biliary Cirrhosis (PBC)

PBC has a strong female preponderance, occurs around the age of 50, cause is unknown. It is characterized by portal inflammation and necrosis of cholangiocytes in small and medium sized bile ducts with cholestatic features including pruritus, jaundice, clay coloured stools; xanthomas, xanthelesma. Extrahepatic causes of cholestasis due to biliary obstruction which can be treated by surgical or endoscopic interventions should be ruled out. Raised levels of serum bilirubin, positive antimitochondrial antibodies (AMA) and liver biopsy showing chronic cholestasis with xanthomatous transformation of the hepatocytes with biliary fibrosis confirm the diagnosis.

Ursodeoxycholic acid (UDCA) is the only approved medical treatment with some degree of efficacy. In decompensated biliary cirrhosis, liver transplant is the treatment of choice.

Primary Sclerosing Cholangitis

It is characterized by primary diffuse inflammation and fibrosis of entire biliary tree resulting into chronic cholestasis where the cause remains unknown. Liver biopsy is not much useful in the diagnosis. Imaging of entire biliary tree is diagnostic. It progresses to biliary cirrhosis.

α1-antitrypsin Deficiency

Alpha 1 antitrypsin (α1AT) is a polypeptide which is an inhibitor of serine proteases in general. Most important targets are neutrophil elastase, cathepsin G and proteinase 3. Homozygous protease inhibitor phenotype (PIZZ) α1 AT deficiency may be discovered at the age of 1–2 months infants because of persistent jaundice. Conjugated bilirubin and serum transaminase levels are mildly or moderately elevated. It gradually progresses to cirrhosis and hepatocellular carcinoma. It is one of the causes of cryptogenic cirrhosis. It is also incriminated in chronic obstructive pulmonary diseases (COPD). Diagnosis is made by demonstrating diminished levels of serum α1 AT.

Drug Induced Liver Injury (DILI)

A large number of drugs have been shown to cause mild (raised serum tranminases) to fatal (acute fulminant hepatitis) liver injury.

Not only drugs used by clinicians but many herbal preparations and dietary supplements cause liver injury.

Environmental factors, biological variations in pharmacokinetics, drug metabolisms and immune response play role in molecular mechanism of liver injury. It is necessary to monitor liver functions while using such drugs and to withdraw them immediately after noticing the injury.

Child-Pugh classification refer to page 33 Table 4.1 of this book.

3

Ascites due to Cirrhosis of the Liver

Alaka Deshpande

Ascites. It can be defined as a pathological accumulation of fluid in the peritoneal cavity.

Pathogenesis. Cirrhosis is characterized by the sinusoidal block. Sinusoidal hypertension is the initial mechanism which causes leak of the fluid in the peritoneal space. It is further contributed by the hypoalbuminaemia which is due to the reduced synthesis of albumin by the liver. Thus, in a portal venous radical it can be schematically depicted that fluid leak as:

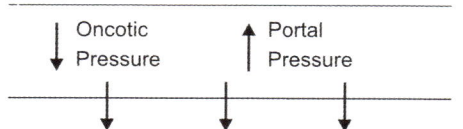

A portal hypertension is defined as a portal venous pressure more than 10 mm of Hg; for the development of ascites a minimal portal pressure gradient of 12 mm of Hg is required.

As the extravascular fluid goes on increasing, the circulating volume decreases which results into avid sodium retention. Urinary sodium excretion is often below 5 mmol/day. Even in the absence of ascites, the normal regulation of sodium balance is lost in cirrhosis.

The vasodilatation theory states that increased production of the vasodilator nitric oxide (NO) is the main cause of vasodilatation. Other vasodilators like adrenomedullin, carbon monoxide, endocannabinoids, prostacyclin, tumour necrosis factors alpha and urotensin are also implicated in the vasodilation of cirrhosis.

Arterial vasodilatation results in the reduction in effective arterial blood volume leading to the activation of renin-angiotensin-aldosterone system (RAAS) which results into retention of sodium and water which further increases the peritoneal leak. In addition to RAAS, Angiotensin II is a potent stimulator for the non-osmotic release of anti-diuretic hormone (ADH). In about a third cirrhotic patients the plasma renin activity is found to be low. In such cases it is proposed that sodium retention occurs unrelated to vasodilatation and the vascular changes are secondary.

In Summary

Ascites in cirrhosis results from:
1. Sinusoidal hypertension and Na$^+$ and water retention (arterial vasodilatation theory), and
2. Overfill theory postulates primary retention of sodium.

Circulation of Ascites

The visceral peritoneum has a large capillary bed through which ascitic fluid constituents are in dynamic equilibrium with the plasma. The ascitic fluid is continuously in circulation, about half leaving and entering the peritoneal cavity every hour.

The rate of reabsorption of ascitic fluid is limited to about 700–900 ml/day.

INVESTIGATIONS

1. Baseline investigations like complete blood count (CBC), complete urine exam, liver function tests including serum glutamic-oxaloacetic transaminase (SGOT), siamane glutamate pyruvate transaminase (SGPT) S. alkaline phosphatase, serum proteins-albumin, globulin, and serum creatinine.
   - S. electrolytes
   - S. prothrombin time, international normalised ratio (INR)

2. Abdominal ultrasonography.
   It is a non-invasive and safe investigation. It reveals:
   A Size of the liver
   In advanced cases of cirrhosis, the liver is small, shrunken, the echogenicity is increased due to fibrosis.
   B Splenomegaly
   C Size of portal vein and collaterals if present
   D Presence of ascites
   F Right hydrothorax
   G Presence of thrombus in portal vein or inferior vena caval (IVC) if any
   H Other organs in the abdomen

3. Ultrasonography (USG) guided paracentesis and/or liver biopsy.

Diagnostic Paracentesis

Diagnostic paracentesis of about 30 ml of ascitic fluid is carried out everytime patient is hospitalized.

Appearance of the fluid—is clear, and straw coloured.

Blood stained fluid may be due to:
   i. Traumatic tap
   ii. Recent paracentesis or
   iii. Invasive investigation such as liver biopsy
   iv. Tuberculosis (common in India)
   v. Malignancy
   vi. Acute/chronic pancreatitis

1. Serum ascites albumin gradient (SAAG)
2. Ascitic proteins

Serum: Ascites albumin gradient (SAAG) are two most useful and inexpensive tests to determine the source of ascites.

a. When the fluid leaks from an inflamed peritoneal surface and/or from the high protein mesenteric lymph as in lymphatic obstruction the total protein content of ascites is more than 2.5 gm/dl, e.g. peritoneal tuberculosis (TB), malignancy. It also happens in post-sinusoidal hypertension.

   In cirrhosis, the protein content of the liver lymph is very low. With sinusoidal collapse or block due to fibrous tissue deposition in the sinusoids as seen in the cirrhosis, the sinusoids are less leaky to macro-molecules so that the protein content of the leaked out fluid is low.

b. Serum ascites albumin gradient (SAAG)—Substraction of ascitic fluid albumin from the serum albumin correlates well with sinusoidal hypertension. The cut-off for SAAG is more than 1.1 gm/dl indicates cirrhosis.
   SAAG
   Cut-off 1.1 gm/dl ascites protein
   Cut-off 2.5 gm/dl
   Cirrhosis high-low
   Cardiac ascites high-high
   Peritoneal TB/malignant low-high

Cell Count of Ascitic Fluid

In ascites due to cirrhosis, the white cell count is less than 100 cells/mm^3 mainly lymphocytes.

Increased white cell count of more than 250 cells/mm^3 predominantly polymorpho-nuclear cells indicate infective/inflammatory response indicating subacute bacterial peritonitis (SBP). Ascitic fluid LDH is raised in SBP.

Ascitic fluid culture may be indicated if infection is suspected.

Differential diagnosis of ascites:
   1. *Malignant ascites*
   2. *Peritoneal tuberculosis*
   3. *Congestive heart failure:* Diagnostic points are raised jugular venous pressure, hepatomegaly, oedema feet and presence

of cardiac lesion. Oedema feet appears before ascites.

4. *Constrictive pericarditis:* Raised jugular venous pressure (JVP), paradoxical pulse, CHF and 2-D echo evidence.

5. *Chylous ascites:* Milky white ascitic fluid suggests chylous ascites. Increased levels of chylomicrons are seen. Ascitic fluid triglycerides content is > 200 mg/dl. The most common cause is post-surgical lymyhatic disruption. In India, rarely it could be due to chronic microfilarial infection blocking lymphatics.

6. *Meigs' syndrome:* Ovarian cyst with ascites with right sided hydrothorax are the components of this syndrome.

Natural history of cirrhotic ascites

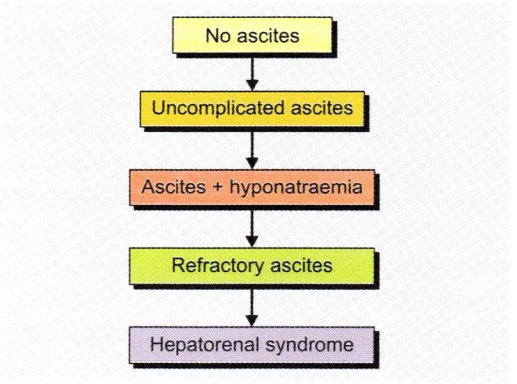

Management of Cirrhotic Ascites

Baseline liver function tests and renal function tests along with serum electrolytes should be determined.

Restriction of Sodium Intake

Dietary sodium has to be restricted to 70–90 mmol/day, i.e. 1.5–2 gms/day, no added salt.

DIURETICS

Spironolactone

a. Initial dose of spironolactone (aldosterone antagonist) is 50–100 mg/day depending upon severity of ascites. If body weight loss is less than 0.5 kg/day the dose of spironolactone can be increased every 4th day by 100 mg while keeping a check on serum creatinine and potassium. If inadequate response on 4th day or there is hyperkalaemia, a loop diuretic like frusemide 40 mg/day is added.

b. Combination of spironolactone + frusemide may be started with close monitoring of laboratory parameters.

c. Diuretics should be stopped if patient develops hypokalaemia, azotemia or 'wing flap' tremors.

Daily weight chart is maintained. Maximum daily weight loss of 0.5 kg/day (1 kg/day in patient with oedema feet) is indicative of response to diuretics.

Paracentesis

In a case of tense ascites causing respiratory embarrassment or IVC compression, therapeutic paracentesis should be carried out with due precaution. Removal of a large amount of ascitic fluid at a time results into a loss of 5 to 10 gm of proteins per litre. Total paracentesis may cause sudden hypovolaemia leading to hypotension and renal failure (Post-paracentesis circulatory syndrome).

It may also result into electrolyte imbalance.

It may precipitate hepatic encephalopathy.

Albumin replacement is more effective in preventing post-paracentesis hypovolaemia and hyponatraemia.

Refractory Ascites

It is defined as ascites not responding to salt restriction and maximum dose of diuretics in hospitalised patient under supervision. The failure of response is indicated by minimal or no weight loss despite higher dose of diuretics or development of complications of diuretic therapy. It has been reported in <10% of cirrhotic patients.

Therapeutic paracentesis: Before undertaking the paracentesis, colloid replacement is necessary. Studies recommend human albumin infusion of 10 gm per litre of ascitic fluid removal. After removal of 5 litres of fluid albumin infusion is optional, one may infuse albumin 5 gm/litre of fluid removal.

Transjugular intrahepatic portosystemic shunts (TIPS): TIPS has become the main second line option in refractory ascites in cirrhosis. TIPS can convert diuretic resistant ascites to diuretic sensitive ascites. It is a challenging procedure carried out by the interventional radiologist.

- Criteria for TIPS
- Age < 65 yrs.
- Child-Pugh score >12
- Models of endstage liver disease* (MELD) score >18
- Left ventricular ejection fraction (LVEF) > 60%
- No alcoholic hepatitis
- Facility to monitor mental status and lactulose administration
- Model for end stage liver disease
- TIPS—Transjugular intrahepatic porto-systemic shunt.

It is a stenting procedure carried out by interventional radiologist best performed under general anaesthesia but can be done under sedation and local anaesthesia.

The internal jugular vein is punctured to pass a cannula into the hepatic vein, usually the middle right vein. A track needs to be created between the hepatic and the portal vein. Under the ultrasonographic guidance a needle puncture of the portal vein is made, this track is ballooned and self-expanding metal stent covered by polytetrafluroethylene (PTFE) is placed through the track.

The spontaneous bacterial peritonitis (SBP) should be treated with third generation cephalosporins administered intravenously for 5–7 days.

Hepatorenal Syndrome

Development of renal failure in absence of identifiable renal pathology in a patient with severe liver disease is hepatorenal syndrome. It is potentially a reversible syndrome. It is functional renal failure rather than a structural disturbance in renal functions.

Mechanism: It is not fully understood, but the impaired renal functions are thought to result from the severest form of vascular and neurohumoral changes associated with severe liver disease. It is a direct result of haemodynamic derangement and cardiovascular changes of liver cirrhosis.

Portal hypertension is an initiator of haemodynamic changes in cirrhosis. There is increasing resistance to portal inflow. Changes in shear stress of the portal vessel wall lead to production of various vasodilators such as nitric oxide, CO, endogenous cannabinoids in portal circulation. The splanchnic vascular bed is dialated leading to reduction in the effective arterial volume. One of the effects of reduction in effective arterial blood volume is activation of various vasoconstrictor systems. These includes renin-angiotensin-aldosterone (RAS) system, sympathetic nervous system and the non-osmotic release of vasopressin. Since the renal circulation is particularly sensitive to the effects of various vasoconstrictors. There is decrease in renal blood flow with reduction in glomerular filtration rate (GFR). The reduction in GFR increases intra-renal production of various intrarenal vasoconstrictors such as angiotensin II, adenosine and endothelins causing further deterioration of the renal function. Changes in renal auto-regulation in advanced cirrhosis also contribute to further renal dysfunction.

Abnormal cardiac function in cirrhosis. The hyperdynamic circulation in cirrhosis is thought to be compensatory mechanisms in response to the decreased vascular resistance to maintain haemodynamics. But in advanced cirrhosis further reduction in vascular resistance may not be met with increased cardiac output. This is known as "systolic incompetence". It is now recognized as a part of syndrome called cirrhotic cardiomyopathy which includes diastolic dysfunction and electrophysiologic abnormalities. Recent studies indicate a correlation between low cardiac output, low mean arterial pressures, low renal blood flow contributing the renal functional derangement. No specific clinical features are present, but laboratory parameters reveal rising creatinine. Regular monitoring is required.

Diagnostic criteria are:

1. Cirrhosis with ascites
2. Serum creatinine >1.5 mg/dL
3. No improvement in serum creatinine 2 days after withdrawal of diuretics
4. No improvement in serum creatinine after volume expansion with intravenous albumin [1 gm/kg/d for 3 days; maximum 100 gm]
5. No use of any nephrotoxic agents
6. Absence of shock
7. Absence of kidney disease indicated by <500 mg/d proteinuria or microhaematuria <50 cells/hpf or any ultrasonographic abnormalities of kidneys.

Management

1. Supportive-treat the precipitating cause like infection, GI bleed.
2. Remove nephrotoxic drugs.
3. Measure central venous pressure (CVP)—normal or increased indicates that the cause of acute kidney injury (AKI) is not volume related.
4. Since effective circulatory volume contributes to pathogenesis of HRS, it is necessary to replenish with colloids. Albumin in doses 1 gm/kg/d; max-100 gm/d is given for the same.
5. Haemodiafiltration in case of excessive fluid overload, acidemia, hyperkalaemia.
6. Vasoconstrictors are needed to reverse the splanchnic vasodialatation. Terlipressin in doses 0.5–2 mg every 4–5 hours; noradrenaline 1–3 mg/hr intravenous drip; octreotide + midodrine 100–200 mcg subcutaneously every 8 hours and 7.5–12.5 mg orally thrice daily respectively is very effective.
7. Liver transplantation.

4

Portal Hypertension

Alaka Deshpande

PORTAL SYSTEM OF CIRCULATION

It is a system of circulation where the veins begin from the venous end of capillaries and end in capillaries.

In systemic circulation, the capillary circulation has two ends, an arteriolar end and venous end.

1. The arteriole ends in capillaries. The arterioles carry oxygenated blood and nutrients which through capillaries are supplied to the tissues for metabolism and production of energy.
2. The CO_2 and other toxic materials produced as a result of tissue metabolism are carried by the venous end of the capillary circulation.

These capillaries form venules which join to form bigger veins which drain into the vena cava. Thus, ultimately deoxygenated blood reaches the right side of the heart.

But in portal circulation the veins which begin from capillaries, end in capillaries.

There are two sites of portal system of circulation in the body:

1. **Hypothalamo-hypophyseal circulation:** The hormone releasing factors released from the hypothalamus are absorbed in the venous end of the capillaries. These factors are carried to the pituitary by a portal venous system which ends into capillaries in the pituitary gland.

Thus, the hormone releasing factors from the hypothalamus directly reach the pituitary gland without entering the systemic circulation where they may be degraded. Pituitary is finally drained by the systemic veins.

2. **Portal circulation between gastrointestinal tract including pancreas, spleen and the liver:** The GI tract, pancreas, and spleen are drained by veins which begin from the capillaries. Instead of opening into vena cava, these veins join to form a portal vein which ends into capillaries in the liver, e.g. after assimilation of food, the veins of the intestines will have very high levels of glucose, amino acids, etc. which are carried to the liver by portal vein. The hepatocytes extract the excess glucose and other nutrients and store them. Finally, the liver is drained by the hepatic vein which opens into inferior vena cava just before the IVC enters the right atrium. Thus, portal circulation safeguards normoglycaemia in a systemic circulation.

Portal Vein

The superior mesentric vein and the splenic vein join to form a 'portal vein' which enters the liver at porta hepatis, divides into two main branches right and left supplying blood to each lobe (Fig. 4.1). The portal blood flow in man is about 1000–1200 ml/min.

Superior mesentric vein (SMV). The tributaries from the intestines, colon, head of the pancreas and from the stomach via right gastroepiploic vein form the superior mesenteric vein.

Splenic vein. About 5–15 channels in splenic hilum drain the spleen. These together with left gastroepiploic vein, tributaries from the head of the pancreas form splenic vein which is joined by inferior mesenteric vein which drains left part of the colon and rectum.

The O_2 content of portal venous blood is less only by 1.9 volumes per cent compared to the arterial blood. In other words, the metabolic activity and O_2 demand by GI tract being much less (except after meals) the portal venous blood is much less deoxygenated compared to the systemic veins.

LIVER CIRCULATION

The liver receives blood from:

1. *Hepatic artery.* Less than one-third of the blood supply of the liver comes from the hepatic artery (Fig. 4.2). It is oxygenated blood, coming under the arterial pressure which is higher compared to the portal venous pressure.

2. *Portal vein.* More than two-thirds of the blood supply of the liver is from the portal vein.

   - It is at a lower pressure compared to the hepatic artery.
   - O_2 saturation is almost like an arterial blood.
   - It has a high content of the digested food products.
   - Low pressure and high O_2 saturation facilitates the uptake of various food products like glucose, amino acids, by the hepatocytes.
   - The ammonia produced by colonic organisms and other toxic products brought to the liver are detoxified by the liver.

Finally, the liver is drained by the hepatic vein.

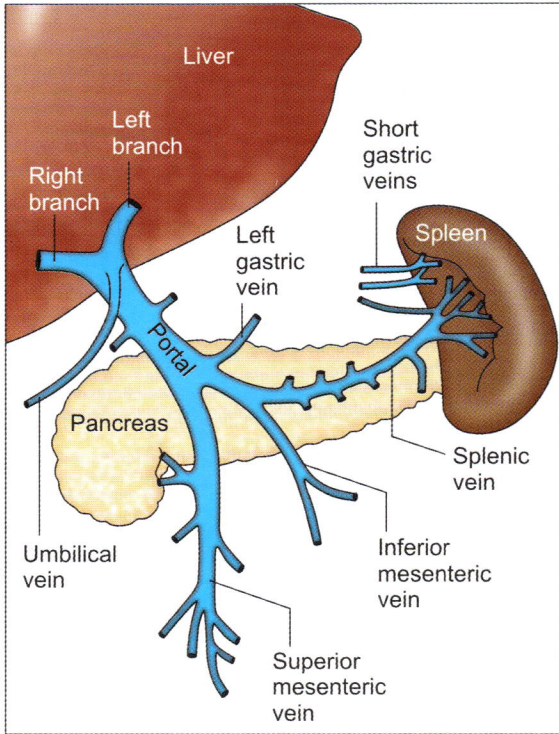

Fig. 4.1: The anatomy of the portal venous system. The portal vein is posterior to the pancreas.

Vessel	Flow	Pressure
Portal vein	1200 ml/min	7 mm of Hg
Hepatic artery	400 ml/min	100 mm of Hg
Hepatic vein	1600 ml/min	4 mm of Hg

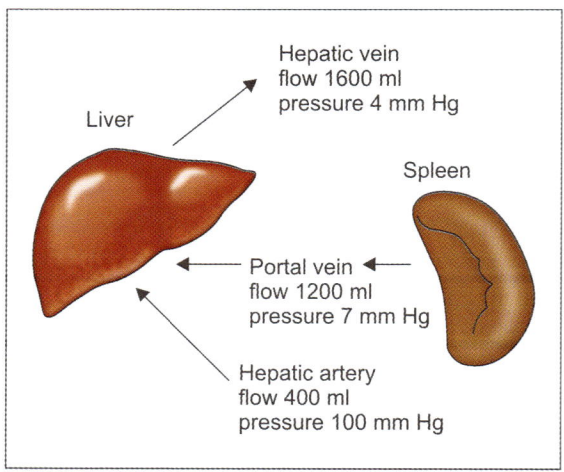

Fig. 4.2: Liver circulation

PORTAL HYPERTENSION (PHT)

The portal venous pressure is normally 7 mm of Hg. When the portal pressure increases to more than 10 mm of Hg it indicates portal hypertension.

However, all patients with raised portal pressure need not show the signs of PHT. A high intra-abdominal pressure due to pregnancy or meteorism increases both portal as well as inferior vena caval (IVC) pressure but produces no signs of PHT because it does not change pressure gradient. Therefore, it is customary to express measurements of portal pressure as the gradient between portal and IVC pressure, i.e. portal pressure gradient.

The signs/complications of PHT are observed when the pressure gradient is raised above the threshold value of 12 mm Hg. This defines what is clinically significant PHT.

Pathophysiology of Portal Hypertension

Portal pressure = Portal inflow × Outflow resistance

PHT is caused by two simultaneously occurring haemodynamic processes.

1. Increased outflow resistance to the portal blood flow is due to:
   a. Collapse of reticulin framework of the liver with distortion of hepatic architecture with sinusoidal collapse.
   b. Extensive fibrosis.
   c. Nodular transformation compressing venous radicals.
2. Increased portal venous inflow due to vasodilatation in the splanchnic vascular bed:
   - Related to endothelial dysfunction.
   - Reduced bioavailability of nitric oxide (NO) molecules.
   - Splanchnic arteriolar vasodilatation which is multifactorial.
   - Glucagon is a humoral vasodilator and elevated levels of glucagon are observed in cirrhotics.

- Endocannabinoids, prostaglandins, and carbon monoxide have been incriminated for vasodilatation.

Portosystemic collateral circulation which develops with portal hypertension is also responsible for the dilatation and hypertrophy of pre-existing vascular channels.

The collateral circulation may carry as much as 90% of the blood entering in the portal system. The vascular resistance of these vessels become the major component of overall resistance to portal blood flow.

Normally, about 100% of the portal venous blood flow can be recovered from the hepatic vein whereas in cirrhosis only 13% is recovered.

Sites of Portosystemic Collaterals

When the portal circulation is obstructed either within or outside the liver, a remarkable collateral circulation develops to carry portal blood into the systemic veins. Formation of collaterals is a complex process involving the opening, dilatation, and hypertrophy of pre-existing vascular channels. Collaterals develop in response to increased portal pressure.

Sites of Portosystemic Collateral Circulation

1. At the cardia of the stomach where the protective squamous epithelium adjoins the absorptive columnar epithelium: left gastric vein, posterior gastric, short gastric veins of the portal system anastomose with the intercostals, diaphragmo-esophageal and azygos minor veins of the caval system—These are oesophageal and gastric varices.
2. Superior haemorrahoidal veins of the portal system anastomose with the middle and inferior haemorrahoidal veins of the caval system at the anus. These are haemorrhoids.
3. The relics of paraumbilical veins of fetal umbilical circulation open up in the falciform ligament with the abdominal wall veins of the caval system, e.g. dilated tortuous epigastric vein, and caput medusae.

4. Where the abdominal organs are in contact with the abdominal wall or retroperitoneal tissue:
   i. Bare area of the liver to the diaphragm,
   ii. Omentum and spleno-renal ligament.
5. Splenic vein to the left renal vein.

The development of portosystemic collaterals is a complex process which involves the following of the pre-existing vascular channels.

1. Opening
2. Dilatation, and
3. Hypertrophy

Collaterals develop in response to increased portal pressure. A minimum threshold of hepatic venous pressure gradient (HVPG) of 10 mm Hg should be reached.

$$HVPG = WHVP - FHVP$$

(WHVP–Wedged hepatic venous pressure, FHVP free hepatic venous pressure)

The development of portosystemic collaterals is also influenced by vascular cell endothelial growth factor (VEGF) dependant angiogenic process.

Manipulation of VEGF may be of therapeutic value.

Etiology of the Portal Hypertension

Obstruction to the outflow of the portal venous blood is the main cause of PHT. PHT is the sequelae of the cirrhosis.

In clinical medicine cirrhosis is the most common cause of PHT. In cirrhosis there is obstruction at the level of sinusoids. Hence the aetiology can be classified as:

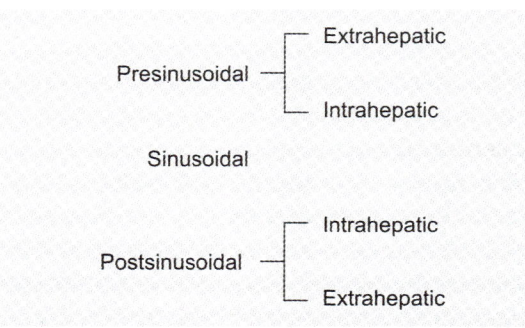

Extrahepatic Presinusoidal

- Thrombosis of the portal vein in neonatal period.
- Pylephlebitis secondary to intra-abdominal sepsis, acute appendicitis, acute peritonitis, sepsis.
- Extension of fibrosis of the umbilical vein.
- Hepatic arterio-venous malformations. A–V malformations, angiomatosis
- Thrombosis of portal vein, splenic vein or superior mesenteric vein
- Hypercoagulable states
- Hetero/homozygous deficiency states of protein C, protein S
- Other prothrombotic conditions
  - Antithrombin III
  - Myeloproliferative disorders which may be latent
  - Prothrombin gene mutation G20210A
- Traumatic-vehicular accidents
- Post-operative particularly post-splenectomy
- Ulcerative colitis, Crohn's disease may be complicated by PV thrombosis
- It may be secondary to primary sclerosing cholangitis
- Polycythemia rubra vera
- Rarely associated with pregnancy, with use of oral contraceptives
- Thrombophlebitis migrans particularly in older women
- Retroperitoneal fibrosis
- Behçet's disease
- Compression of portal vein at porta hepatis
  - Hepatocellular carcinoma
  - Carcinoma of the pancreas (chronic pancreatitis is frequently associated with splenic vein thrombosis)
  - Metastatic deposits in the lymph nodes at porta hepatis, e.g. lymphoma, chronic lymphocytic leukaemia, etc.
  - Tuberculosis, sarcoidosis.

Intrahepatic Presinusoidal

- Schistosomiasis
- Congenital portal fibrosis

- Rarely primary biliary cirrhosis
- Sarcoidosis
- Toxins like vinyl chloride, arsenic, and copper
- Hypervitaminosis A
- Amyloidosis

Sinusoidal

Cirrhosis of the liver.

Intrahepatic Post-sinusoidal

Veno-occulusive disease

Extrahepatic Post-sinusoidal

- Veno-occulusive disease
- Constrictive pericarditis (rare)
- IVC obstruction (rare)

Portal vein occlusion is particularly common in India accounting for 20–30% of all variceal bleeding.

In about half of the patients the cause of the portal hypertension remains obscure. Some of these cases are associated with autoimmune disorders such as rheumatoid arthritis, pernicious anaemia, hypothyroidism, and diabetes.

PRIMARY PORTAL HYPERTENSION

In past, cases of malaria and *kala azar* in tropical countries used to develop massive splenomegaly due to paucity of effective therapies against these infections.

The splenic enlargement used to be massive reaching almost to right iliac fossa. It is also known as tropical splenomegaly. By the shear size of the spleen, the venous return from the spleen is markedly increased. Over the years this increased venous return resulted into sclerotic changes in the splenic vein thus raising the vascular resistance and portal venous pressure.

The PHT in these cases is not severe, variceal bleed is a rarity. This is a extrahepatic presinusoidal cause of PHT.

Splenomegaly is a sign of portal hypertension but in this case splenomegaly is the cause of portal hypertension.

Clinical Features

Clinical features related to are as follows:
Portal hypertension
a. Splenomegaly
b. Portosystemic collaterals
c. Signs of decompensated cirrhosis of the liver
d. Chronic hepatic encephalopathy.

The most common cause of PHT is cirrhosis of the liver. Due to sinusoidal block, there is increased backflow in portal system which results in:

a. **Splenomegaly:** Usually, there is moderate splenomegaly up to umbilicus. If **splenomegaly** is not detected ultrasonography of the abdomen reveals splenic enlargement in early stages. Usually, there is moderate splenomegaly up to umbilicus. The size may vary depending on the treatment of PHT or after hematemesis.

The patient may complain of a lump in the left hypochondrium. He may get dragging pain in LHC due to splenomegaly. He may complain of fullness of the stomach after small meals.

A moderate splenomegaly may cause signs and symptoms due to hypersplenism.

Congestive gastropathy: Portal hypertensive or congestive gastropathy results from congestion of GI mucosa due to back pressure. Patient complains of nausea, fullness or bloating of the stomach even with small meals. Upper GI scopy reveals the changes mainly in the antrum and fundus of the stomach. Mosaic like pattern of mucosa in noted along with red pointed lesions which predict high-risk for bleeding. Intramucosal haemmorhage may be noted as black, brown spots (Fig. 4.3).

Portal hypertensive colonopathy may be present in half of the patients which can be diagnosed on colonoscopy.

b. **Portosystemic collaterals:** Clinical examination may show dilated and tortuous veins of the anterior abdominal wall. Particularly an epigastric vein may be noted with patient in a standing position. It is dilated and tortuous.

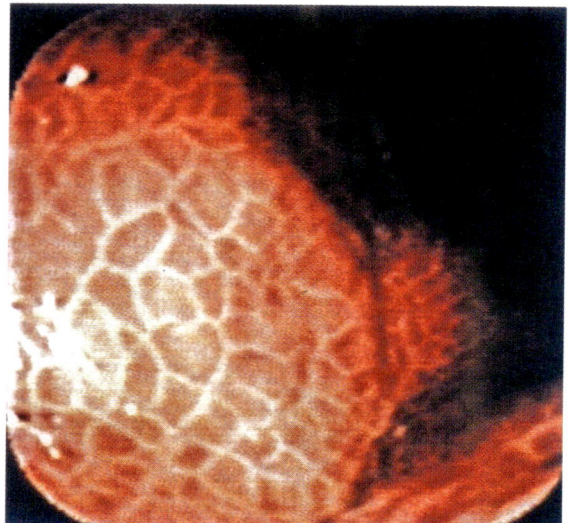

Fig. 4.3: Portal gastropathy. A mosaic of red and yellow is seen together with petechial haemorrhages.

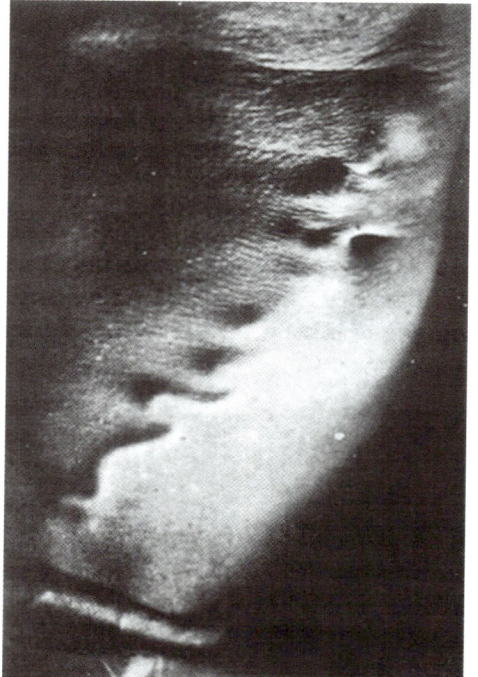

Fig. 4.4: An anterior abdominal wall vein in a patient with cirrhosis of the liver

Caput medusae. Veins on anterior abdominal wall radiating from the umbilicus are termed as caput medusae. (Fig. 4.5 a and b).

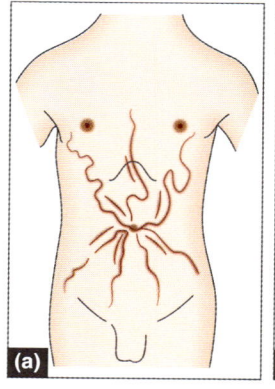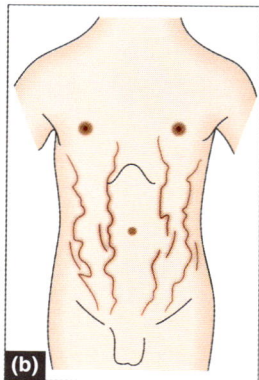

Fig. 4.5a and b: (a) Caput medusae, and (b) Direction of the blood flow

Normally, the direction of the blood flow in the veins of anterior abdominal wall is away from the umbilicus.

In presence of portal hypertension the direction of the blood flow does not change.

If there is reversal of the direction of blood flow it suggests thrombosis of respective vena cava, e.g. Veins below the umbilicus drain in the inferior vena cava (IVC), the direction of blood flow is away from the umbilicus, i.e. from umbilicus downwards towards symphysis pubis. If the direction of the blood flow in these veins is reversed, i.e. from below upwards, it indicates IVC obstruction. Same is true for veins above the umbilicus.

A thrill due to increased blood flow may be palpable over larger veins. A venous hum may be heard.

Cruveilheir-Baumgarten syndrome: A loud venous hum is heard at the umbilicus due to congenital patency of the umbilicus vein communicating to the veins of anterior abdominal wall.

Esophageal varices: As discussed earlier, dilated tortuous veins are seen on endoscopy in the oesophagus. Commonly there are four columns of the blood, varicosity is graded according to the severity as mild grade I to severe grade IV.

The severe tortuosity may lead to bleeding and patient presents with hematemesis.

In addition to oesophageal varices, varices are seen in the gastric fundus.

With hematemesis a large amount of the blood from bleeding varices goes down the GI tract and cause melaena. Hematemesis may precipitate hepatic encephalopathy.

Rectum. Anorectal varices are seen on sigmoidoscopy and may cause bleeding per rectum.

c. **Signs of decompensated cirrhosis of liver:** These are present like spider naevi, gynaecomastia, jaundice, ascites, etc. (Refer to Chapter 1).

d. **Chronic Hepatic encephalopathy** (Refer to Chapter 5).

The liver size and consistency may be noted. Firm liver supports cirrhosis while soft liver suggests extra hepatic PHT. Smaller the liver severe is the cirrhosis.

Investigations

1. For liver functions
   Liver function tests
2. For portal hypertension
   a. Visualization of portal vein
   b. Measurement of portal pressure

   a. **Visualization of the portal system**
      – Radiography
      – Endoscopy
      – Imaging

Radiography. Barium swallow shows presence of varices as filling defects in the regular contour of the oesophagus. Presently it is replaced by upper GI endoscopy.

Upper GI endoscopy. It is a safe noninvasive technique to directly visualize the oesophagus and the stomach-duodenum. Varices are seen as longitudinal tortuous and dilated venous columns. The number of varices, length and severity may be recorded.

Varices in the fundus of the stomach must be looked for. Endoscopy of the stomach may reveal portal hypertensive gastropathy.

Imaging

1. **Abdominal ultrasonography:** It is a safe noninvasive technique which may show:
   a. Splenomagely
   b. Size and echogenicity of the liver
   c. Portal vein and superior mesentric veins, the diameters of these vessels are measured.
   d. Collateral vessels may be seen in the splenic hilum, and along the stomach.
   e. Presence of thrombosis in the portal vein may be seen as an echogenic area.
   f. A–V malformations or angiomatous malformations may be noted in the porta hepatis.
   g. Presence of ascites.
   h. Doppler ultrasound can be used to study the flow pattern.
2. **Magnetic resonance angiography:** MR angiography is more reliable than the Doppler ultrasound. It detects portal patency, flow velocity, morphology, etc. Portal venography may be indicated if surgical treatment of PHT is contemplated.

Measurement of Portal Pressure

Hepatic venous pressure gradient (HVPG)— A balloon catheter is introduced into the femoral or internal jugular vein and under fluoroscopic control it is advanced to the hepatic vein.

Two measurements are taken namely:
1. Wedged hepatic venous pressure (WHVP)— It is a measurement of a hepatic sinusoidal pressure.
2. Free hepatic venous pressure (FHVP)— It is measured by inflating and deflating the balloon in the tip of the catheter.

$$HVPG = WHVP–FHVP$$

The normal values of HPVG are up to 5 mm of Hg.

The most common cause of PHT is sinusoidal block therefore HVPG is a good indicator. It has been shown that critical thresh-hold for formation of varices is HPVG of 10 mm of Hg and that for the appearance of other complications such as variceal bleed, ascites, etc. is 12 mm of Hg.

A recent study has shown that HPVG of < 10 mm of Hg has a 90% probability of not developing clinical decompensation in a median follow-up of 4 years.

The limitation of HPVG is that it does not reflect portal pressure in cases of PHT due to presinusoidal causes.

The PHT due to post-sinusoidal causes show increase in both WHVP and FHVP with a normal range of HPVG.

Hepatic vein catheterization is useful for evaluation of PHT.

To monitor response to pharmacological agents, e.g. β-blockers.

For prognostic evaluation during variceal bleed.

To assess progression of chronic liver disease.

Specific Investigations for cause of PHT. If the cause of the PHT is not detected by imaging then specific investigations to ascertain the same may be carried out. Since the most common cause of PHT is cirrhosis it is discussed in detail.

Management of Portal Hypertension

Variceal bleeding is associated with progressive decline in survival following first episode. It is also associated with high morbidity and mortality. It may be acute hematemesis or chronic ooze resulting into melaena. It may cause iron deficiency anaemia due to chronic blood loss. Bleeding varices may have deleterious effects on the liver function due to

- Diminished oxygen supply to hepatocytes
- Release of cytokines
- Increased protein catabolism raising metabolic demands
- Fall in blood pressure resulting in diminished hepatic arterial flow on which the regenerating nodules depend.

- In acute hematemesis, a large amount of blood goes down the intestines. Increased production and absorption of ammonia/ nitrogen from the gut may precipitate hepatic encephalopathy.

The key objective in the management of PHT in cirrhosis is primary prevention of variceal bleed.

All cirrhotic patients should undergo an endoscopic examination as a part of their evaluation along with liver function tests. Patient should be assessed as per Child-Pugh classification (Table 4.1).

Patient should abstain from alcohol. Aspirin and NSAIDS should be avoided.

Non-selective β-blockers like propranolol or nadalol are used. No data currently exists about its utility in case of gastric varices.

Band ligation of varices is recommended in primary prevention of variceal bleed.

Combination therapy with ligation or other drugs has no added advantage and hence is not recommended.

Endoscopic sclerotherapy Injection of sclerosant substance in varices results into obliteration of varices. However, it requires skilled endoscopist. Sclerotherapy is also associated with 10–20% complications like bleeding, ulceration, stenosis. β-blockers alone are shown to be superior to sclerotherapy.

Transjugular intrahepatic portosystemic shunts (TIPS) Current data does not recommend TIPS for primary prevention of variceal haemmorhage.

Four prospective randomized trials comparing surgical portocaval shunts with medical therapy over 25 years concluded that surgical procedures are not recommended for primary prevention of variceal bleed.

Clinical Management of Active Variceal Haemmorhage

Depending on the blood loss, patient may be haemodynamically unstable as manifested by

- Hypotension

Table 4.1: Child-Pugh classification			
Group designation	A	B	C
Serum bilirubin (mg/dL)	Below 2.0	2.0–3.0	Over 3.0
Serul albumin (g/dL)	Over 3.5	3.0–3.5	Under 3.0
Ascites	None	Easily controlled	Poorly controlled
Neurological disorder	None	Minimal	Advanced coma
Nutrition	Excellent	Good	Poor: Wasting

*1 mg = 17 µmol/L.

- Fall in hematocrit (3 gm drop in haemoglobin is 9% drop in hematocrit)
- Aspiration pneumonia
- Gram-negative infection

The primary goals of management during active bleeding are:

1. Haemodynamic resuscitation
2. Treatment of bleeding
3. Prevention and management of complications

Haemodynamic Resuscitation

The goal is to restore tissue perfusion. Volume replacement with plasma, plasma expanders is advised till the packed cell transfusion is organized. Haemoglobin may be maintained at 8–9 gm%. Care should be taken to avoid volume overload. Urine output should be maintained at least 50 ml/hr. Renal functions are to be monitored.

Pre-existing coagulopathy in a cirrhotic patient needs to be corrected with Inj vitamin K. Transfusion of platelets and fresh frozen plasma may be considered in a case of severe coagulopathy.

Aspiration pneumonia. It complicating the haematemesis usually has a fatal outcome. All patients with massive haematemesis or a case with altered mental status and active bleeding need protection of the airway.

Endotracheal intubation is necessary.

Prophylactic antibiotics are given. Aminoglycosides should be avoided.

About 20% of patients with active bleeding have bacterial infection at the time of hospitalization. UTI, bacterial pneumonias, spontaneous bacterial peritonitis are common and should be treated. Third generation cephalosporins are given immediately.

Mental status should be monitored. Sedation is avoided. Chronic alcoholism being the common cause of cirrhosis with PHT, thiamine is indicated. If delirium tremens are present they should be treated.

Lactulose is given orally or by enema to remove blood from GI tract to prevent encephalopathy. Patient needs to be monitored for electrolytes, acidosis/alkalosis, phosphate levels and blood sugar. Hypophosphatemia is corrected by phosphate enema.

Treatment of Acute Variceal Bleeding

1. Vasoactive drugs
   Vasopressin, terlipressin
2. Mechanical balloon compression
   Sengstaken–Blakemore tube tamponades
3. Endoscopic band ligation/sclerotherapy
4. TIPS

Vasoactive Drugs

Vasopressin directly constricts mesenteric arterioles and decreases portal venous flow. It is given as a continuous infusion of 0.2–0.4 units/min. It should always be accompanied by IV nitroglycerin starting with 40 mcg/min which may be increased up to 400 mcg/min.

Vasopressin may cause coronary vasoconstriction resulting into myocardial, cerebral, bowel ischaemia. Before starting vasopressin, ECG of the patient is taken and during the infusion, cardiac activity may be monitored.

Terlipressin is a long acting vasopressin derivative with lesser side effects. It is a splanchnic vasoconstrictor. It is used as an IV bolus of 2 mg every 4–6 hrs for up to 48 hrs. After an initial control of bleeding (a 24 hour bleeding free period) the dose is halved and maintained for 5 days to prevent early rebleeding. Vasopressin and terlipressin efficacy is comparable however side effects are less and of lesser severity with terlipressin.

Somatostatins. It is a 14 amino acid peptide with properties of inhibiting the growth hormone. It inhibits the release of vasodilator hormone (e.g. glucagon), indirectly causes splanchnic vasoconstriction and reduction in portal inflow.

It has a very short half-life and disappears within minutes after IV bolus.

It is administered as a continuous IV infusion after an initial bolus.

Initial bolus of 250 microgrammes (mcg) followed by IV infusion of 250 mcg/hour.

Infusion may be continued for 5 days.

Octreotide

It is a synthetic somatostatin analog with longer half-life. However, the trial reports are conflicting. Haemodynamic effects of octreotide, the optimal dose and the administrative method have not been established.

It is given as a continuous IV infusion at empiric dosage of 25–50 mcg/hr after an IV bolus of 50 mcg. Treatment duration is 1–5 days. Although the role of octreotide is less well-established it is the current drug of choice in US because of its easy availability compared to somatostatin.

The recent consensus conference summarizes that somatostatin is more effective with fewer side effects than vasopressin. It has therefore replaced vasopressin, as a pharmacological agent of choice to treat active variceal bleed.

Endoscopic treatment It may be

1. *Endoscopic band ligation:* It is used worldwide because of simple technique and effectiveness. A number of randomized control trials (RCT) have established significant benefit of band ligation in the initial treatment of active bleeding compared to sclerotherapy.
2. Endoscopic sclerotherapy requires a skilled endoscopist and the procedure is associated with serious complications in 10–20% of cases.

Balloon tamponade. It is effective in short-term haemostasis. However, it has a high rate of rebleeding as the balloon is deflated. In all these cases airway must be protected. The only role of such treatment is to temporarily stabilize the patient while arranging for a definitive treatment.

TIPS

Transjugular intrahepatic portosystemic shunts can stop bleeding in most patients. However, there are no RCTs. A very high proportion of patients are effectively managed with medical and/or endoscopic therapy. TIPS is confined to rare cases of uncontrolled bleeding which are about less than 10%.

Failure to Control Bleeding

(Baveno IV consensus statement)

The time frame for the acute bleeding episodes should be 120 hr (5 days).

Failure to control the bleeding is defined as

- Fresh haematemesis or nasogastic aspiration of ≥100 mL of fresh blood ≥2 hours after the start of a specific drug treatment or therapeutic endoscopy.
- Development of hypovolemic shock.
- A 3 gm drop in haemoglobin (9% drop of haematocrit) within any 24 hours period if no transfusion is administered. This time frame needs to be further validated.

Flowchart 4.1: Algorithm of management of acute variceal haemorrhage

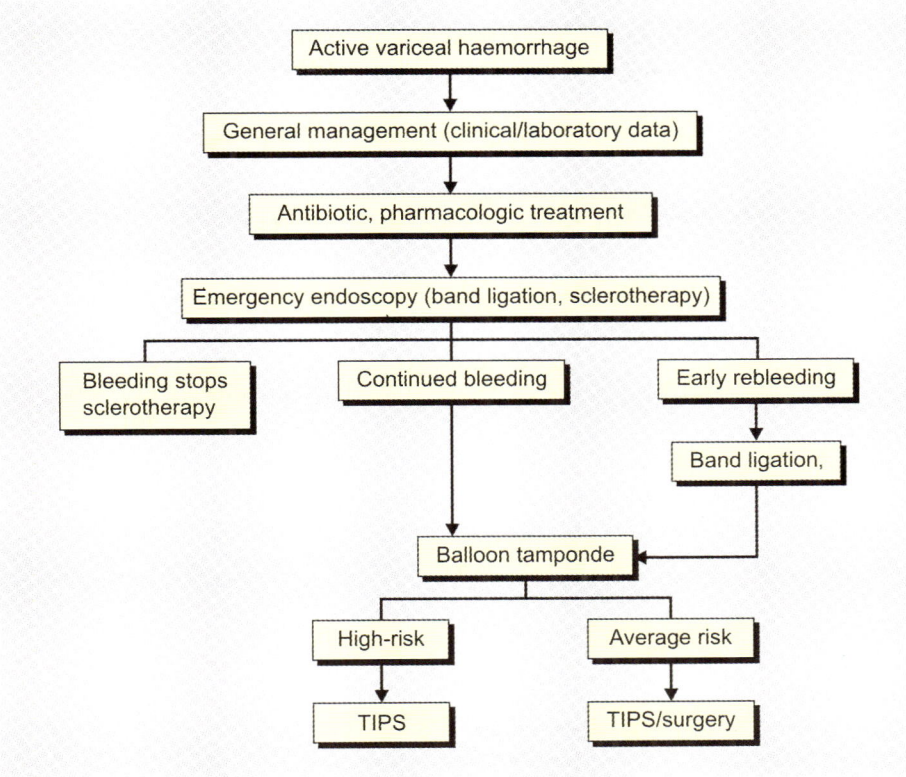

The natural history of an untreated patient who has survived an episode of variceal haemorrhage is characterized by recurrent haemorrhage with consequent liver failure, hepatic encephalopathy, and eventually death (Flowchart 4.1).

"Failure of secondary prophylaxis" is defined as follows:

1. Failure to prevent rebleeding is defined as a single episode of clinically significant rebleeding from portal hypertensive sources after day five.

2. Clinically significant rebleeding is recurrent melena or hematemesis resulting in any of the following:

- Hospital admission
- Blood transfusion
- A 3 gm drop in haemoglobin
- Death within 6 weeks

Many guidelines have shown the best approach in the prevention of recurrent oesophageal variceal bleeding is the combination of non-selective β-blockers plus band ligation.

Surgical Treatment of PHT

After the first episode of variceal bleed, rebleeding occurs in about 70% of cases more so in presence of Child's grade C. Therefore, it is necessary to prevent rebleeding.

Most effective preventive therapy for rebleeding is a combination of repeated endoscopic ligation and non-selective β-blockers.

If TIPS can be placed, surgical portocaval shunts are very rarely performed.

Portocaval Shunts

Portal vein is joined to inferior vena cava either end to side or end to end. The portal venous pressure falls.

Mesocaval shunt is between superior mensenteric vein and inferior vena cava.

Surgical shunts result into fall in hepatic blood flow worsening hepatic functions. 20–40% cases develop chronic hepatic encephalopathy with personality changes.

Myelopathy, paraplegia and cerebellar syndrome are rare.

Currently, with effective pharmacologic agents to reduce the HPVG, and advent of TIPS has successfully treated and prevented rebleeds.

5

Hepatic Encephalopathy

Alaka Deshpande

Hepatic encephalopathy (HE) is the term used to describe a broad range of neurologic and neuropsychiatric impairments seen in patients with significant-underlying liver disease.

Neurological syndromes associated with liver disease have been described as early as hippocrates (460–370 BC) but HE as we know today has been described by Adams and Foley and others in the mid-20th century.

It is characterized by reversible neuro-psychiatric manifestations varying from clinically indiscernible changes in cognition to overt changes in behaviour, intellect, motor functions and consciousness. It is a grave prognostic sign having detrimental effects on the health and survival. It may be episodic or chronic and persistent.

It is seen in:

1. Cirrhosis of liver
2. Acute fulminant hepatitis
3. Chronic portosystemic encephalopathy

Acute hepatitis with hepatic encephalopathy has a very poor prognosis, survival may be about 20%. It is seen in acute fulminant viral hepatitis, alcoholic hepatitis, drug reactions and overdose.

In presence of cirrhosis, the survival is about 70–80%. Various precipitating factors have been responsible for episodic encephalopathy in an otherwise stable cirrhotic. Table 5.1 shows precipitating factors.

Hepatic encephalopathy consensus group in 1998 at the world congress of gastroentrology classified HE as (Flowchart 5.1):

Prior to this meeting HE and portosystemic encephalopathy were interchangably used. Portosystemic encephalopathy indicated that changes in the mental state are mainly because of portosystemic shunts. However, in absence of intrinsic liver disease, it is a rarity. Therefore, the hepatic encephalopathy was classified in three categories as shown in the Table 5.2.

Table 5.1: Precipitating factors	
1. Gastro-intestinal bleeding	7. Diarrhoea/vomiting
2. Sepsis	8. Excessive protein load
3. Hyponatremia	9. Constipation
4. Hypokalaemia	10. Sedatives
5. Abdominal paracentesis	11. Surgical procedure
6. Excessive diuretics	12. TIPS

Flowchart 5.1

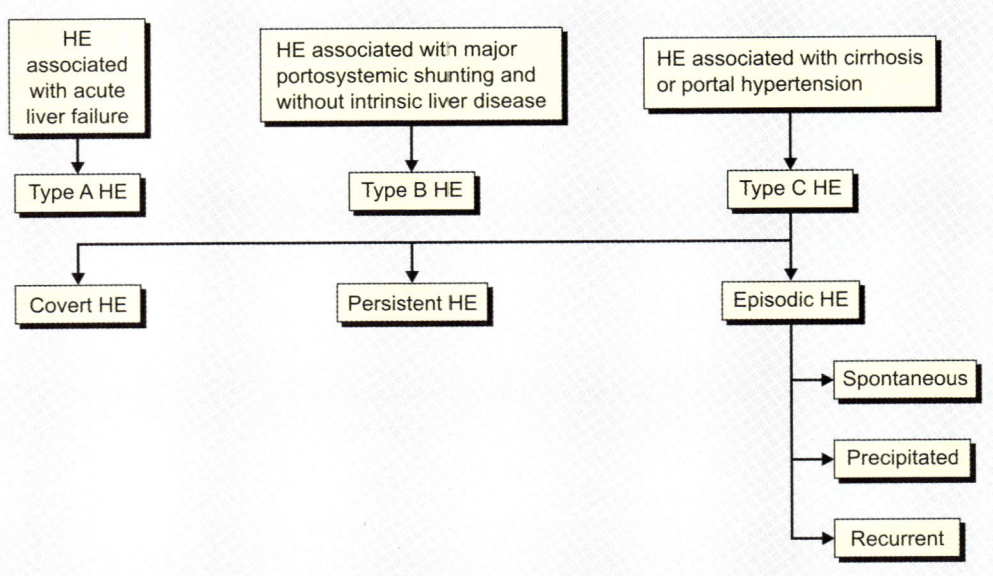

	Table 5.2: Shows the differences in type A HE and type C HE	
	Type A HE	*Type C HE*
Hepatic injury	Acute onset (<8 weeks)	Chronic (at least >6 months)
Animal model	Galactosamine in rabbits/rats	Bile duct ligation and/or carbon tetrachloride in rats
Pathology	Acute hepatoceullar necrosis and hepatic insufficiency	Chronic hepatocellular injury, fibrosis, nodular regeneration and circulatory bypass of the liver
Clinical Profile		
Onset	Acute	Variable: insidious versus acute
Precipitating factors	Uncommon	Common
Cerebral oedema	High-grade edema present	Low-grade edema present
Nutritional state	Normal	Cachexia may be present
Ascites	Absent	Usually present
Portosystemic shunts	Absent	Present
Treatment	Treat cause of liver failure. Usually need liver transplant	Treat precipitating cause along with emipirical therapy
Immediate survival	Low without transplant	High
Persistent neuropsychiatric sequelae after acute episode	No	Prior overt HE patients have worse cognition

Pathogenesis

HE is a syndrome having varied and reversible clinical picture and a multitude of precipitating factors. Therefore, the precise mechanism of the pathogenesis is largely unknown (Fig. 5.1). The key player is hepatocellular dysfunction further contributed by portosystemic shunting of the blood.

Table 5.3: Shows modified West haven criteria to grade HE

Grade	Description	Operative definition
0	No abnormality detected	
Minimal HE	No neurologic symptoms	PHES >2 SD in two or more tests
	Normal clinical examination	ICT >5 lures
	Abnormal psychometric test performance	CF: Critical frequency of 39 Hz or less
		Naming <7 animals in 120 seconds
1	Trivial lack of awareness	Oriented in time and space
	Euphoria or anxiety	
	Shortened attention span	
	Impairment of addition or subtraction	
2	Lethargy or apathy	Disoriented in time (≥3 items incorrect)
	Disorientation for time	Day of the week
	Obvious personality change	Day of the month
	Inappropriate behaviours	The month
		The year
		Oriented in place
3	Somnolence to semi-stupor	Disoriented in place (>2 items incorrect)
	Responsive to stimuli	State/country
	Confused	Region/country
	Gross disorientation	City
	Bizzare behaviour	Place
		Floor/ward
		Disoriented in time, and reduction in Glasgow coma scale (8–14)
4	Coma, unable to test mental state	Unresponsive to painful stimuli (Glasgow coma scale <8)

CF, critical frequency; ICT, inhibitory control test; PHES, psychometric hepatic encephalopathy score; SD, standard deviation.

Portosystemic shunting in the absence of liver dysfunction for example as in the cases of portal vein thrombosis is usually not accompanied by hepatic encephalopathy.

The observation that gut lavage and catharsis results in the resolution of overt hepatic encephalopathy indicates the role of gut derived toxins. The liver as such has a larger role in detoxification. In hepatocellular dysfunction, the gut derived toxins are not detoxified and may gain access to systemic circulation by-passing the liver through portosystemic shunts.

Complex changes follow which directly or indirectly affect the brain function.

Key factors are:

- Gut derived neurotoxins
- Brain water homeostasis
- Oxidative and nitrosative stress
- Infection and inflammation
- Neurotransmitter dysfunction
- Astrocyte dysfunction

Gut derived neurotoxins. Several gut derived neurotoxins are implicated but most important and significant is ammonia.

Normally, ammonia is produced in the gut from:

- Dietary proteins
- Deamination of glutamine
- Bacterial action in the colon

In presence of normal hepatic function the serum ammonia is highly under control as the ammonia from the gut is absorbed by non-ionic diffusion in the portal venous blood

(NH_3 concentration in portal vein is ten times more than systemic arterial concentration).

The extraction of NH_3 by hepatocytes is very high; it is metabolized to urea by urea cycle.

Some ammonia is converted by hepatocytes to glutamine via glutamine synthetase.

The two systems work in harmony keeping hepatic vein NH_4 concentration under tight control.

In cirrhotics the blood NH_4 levels may increase due to:

1. Reduction in functioning hepatocytes
2. Enhanced intestinal absorption of NH_3 due to increased splanchnic blood flow associated with portal hypertension.
3. Bowel colonization by urease containing bacteria
4. Portosystemic shunting
5. Loss of muscle mass resulting into decreased NH_3 metabolism in muscle.

In cirrhotics, although blood brain barrier remains intact, there is greater permeability which increases cerebral ammonia uptake.

The brain has no urea cycle. Ammonia is detoxified by astrocytes through glutamine by glutamine synthetase. NH_3 exerts deleterious effects on the astrocytes, the changes which are referred to as Alzeheimer type II astrocytosis. The changes are most prominent in the cerebral cortex, basal ganglia and thalamus. Ammonia also has a direct effect on the cortical neurons.

Despite these changes, the correlation between circulating blood ammonia concentration and neuropsychiatric changes in hepatic encephalpathy is poor.

Other toxins derived from the gut are mercaptans, indoles, phenols and short and medium chained fatty acids.

Brain Water Homeostasis

The influx of excessive NH_3 in the brain alters the water homeostasis in brain. Osmotically active glutamine accumulates in the astrocytes which results in astrocyte swelling which has significant functional consequences. Other factors like inflammatory cytokines, hyponatremia, benzodiazepine all working synergistically with NH_3 further increase astrocyte swelling.

Oxidative/Nitrosative Stress

The imbalance between production of reactive oxygen/nitric oxide species and their rate of removal results into cell damage and death.

Astrocyte dysfunctions—Several factors cited earlier cause dysfunction of the astrocytes which by various mechanisms cause disruption of glioneuronal communication.

Neurotransmitters

There is a change in multiple neurotransmitters in hepatic encephalopathy with shift in balance between inhibitory and excitatory neurotransmission favouring inhibition.

Infections

Cirrhotics have impaired host defence increasing the vulnerability to infections which frequently precipitate hepatic encephalopathy.

Clinical Features of Hepatic Encephalopathy

A wide spectrum of neuropsychiatric and motor dysfunctions characterize HE. In a known case of cirrohosis with portal hypertension the symptoms can raise a high index of suspicion. HE occurs in decompensated cirrhosis therefore other stigmata of cirrhosis may be present.

Neuropsychiatric Changes

Physical changes. Personality changes, irritability, changed behaviour, apathy, altered sleeping pattern in a cirrhotic should raise the suspicion.

Disturbances in intellectual functions vary from slight impairment to gross confusion.

Constructional apraxia. It is an inability to construct or reproduce simple designs like triangles, stars, etc. Writing is indistinct. A daily signature chart may be maintained.

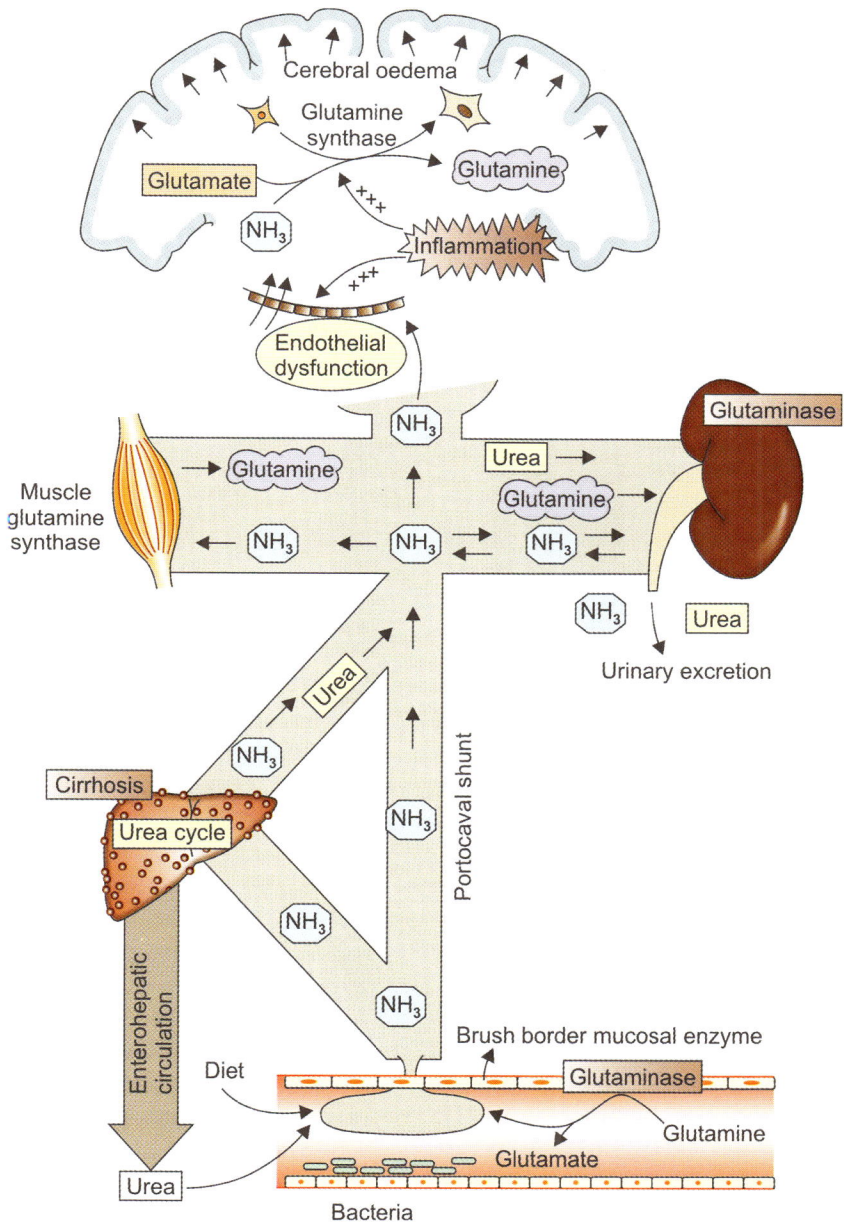

Fig. 5.1: Shows pathogenesis

Motor disturbances include tremors, disorders of speech, rigidity, delayed diadochokinetic movements, astirixis. Deep tendon reflexes may show hypo or hyper-reflexia, plantars may be extensors. Extrapyramidal signs like bradykinesia, rigidity may be present.

Asterixis

It is arrhythmic lapses in the posture. Asterixis is derived from the Greek-α (not) and steraxis (fixed position). It is a failure to actively maintain posture or position. It is elicited by dorsiflexion of the hand with the forearm and fingers extended. The postural

	Table 5.4
Pathogenic factors	*Some proposed mechanism*
Ammonia	Combines with glutamate to form glutamine
	Intracelluar accumulation of glutamine causes astrocyte swelling and cerebral oedema
	Involved in generation of reactive oxygen species (ROS)
Inflammation	Astrocytes and microglial cells release cytokines
	Cytokines affect the integrity of the blood-brain barrier and increase ammonia diffusion into the brain
Neurosteroids	Increased expression of protein 18kDa stimulates neurosteroid synthesis
	Enhances GABAnergic tone by a positive allosteric action on GABA-A receptor
Oxidative and nitrosative stress	Synthesized and released in response to ammonia, inflammatory mediators, hyponatremia, and benzodiazepines
	Has a role in astrocyte swelling and tyrosine nitration of intracellular proteins
Manganese	Preferential accumulation in basal ganglia in cirrhotics with extensive portosystemic shunts
	Has role in formation of type II Alzheimer cells, stimulating neurosteroid synthesis and increasing GABAnergic tone

(GABA, γ-aminobutyric acid)

Table 5.5: Concomitant causes of encephalopathy

- Respiratory failure: hypoxia and hypercapnia
- Gross electrolyte abnormalities
- Status epilepticus or postictal state
- Renal failure and uremia
- Cerebrovascular accident/stroke
- Hypoglycemia
- Central nervous system infections
- Intracerebral/intracranial haemorrhage
- Metabolic acidosis
- Drug intoxication
- Cerebral oedema/intracranial hypertension
- Wernicke-Korsakoff syndrome
- Delirium tremens
- Pancreatic encephalopathy

Table 5.6: Other causes of flapping tremors

- Renal failure
- Respiratory failure
- Severe heart failure
- Hypomagnesemia
- Phenytoin intoxication

lapse causes series of rapid involuntary flexion-extension movements of the wrist called as 'hepatic flap'. The tremors appear like birds flapping their wings (wing flap tremors) (Fig. 5.2).

Diagnosis

Different techniques are used to assess various dysfunctions.

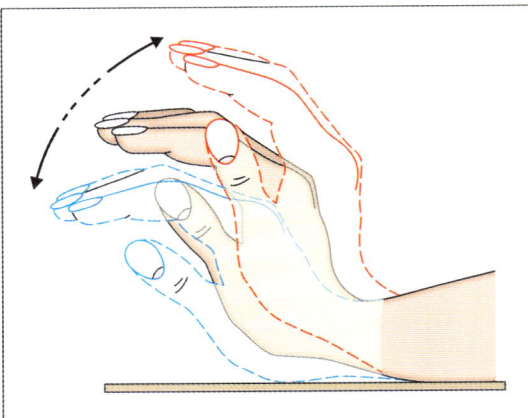

Fig. 5.2: 'Flapping' tremor elicited by attempted dorsiflexion of the wrist with the forearm fixed.

1. Mental status assessment
   - Glasgow coma scale
   - West haven criteria
2. Psychometric testing
3. Electroencephalography EEG
4. Evoked potentials • sensory
   - congnitive
5. Neuroimaging—CT, MRI
   MR spectroscopy

EEG gives evidence of metabolic encephalopathy.
- Slowing of normal alpha frequency
- Triphasic waves or arrhythmic delta activity

Blood Ammonia

The newer techniques to measure blood ammonia are more accurate and are of diagnostic help particularly if the patient is not a known cirrhotic.

Management

Management of HE consists of
1. Supportive care of a patient with altered sensorium
2. Prompt identification and treatment of precipitating factors
3. Treat concomitant conditions (Table 5.5)
4. Empiric therapy of HE (Table 5.7)

1. Patient with severe HE is hospitalized in the intensive care, electively intubated. Most common precipitating factor in

Table 5.7: Empirical therapy for hepatic encephalopathy treatment

- Lactulose 15–30 mL PO two to three times a day titrated to two to three soft bowel movements
- Rifaximin 550 mg PO twice daily
- Neomycin 500 mg PO four times daily (caution in renal failure and in high doses)
- Metronidazole 250 mg PO four times daily (only for short-term use)
- Vancomycin 250 mg PO four times daily
- Sodium benzoate 5 g PO twice daily
- Flumazenil 1–3 mg intravenous (short-lasting therapy)

cirrhotics is upper GI bleed. Aspiration is the greatest risk; so patient is electively intubated. Secondly, a nasogastric tube is passed and stomach lavage is given in case of GI bleed.

Later on the nasogastric (NG) tube may be used for feeding purpose.

Treatment of precipitating factors

Prompt identification of precipitating factors is necessary so that appropriate corrective measures can be taken. In some patients more than one factor may be present. Correction of precipitating factors alone results into 80–90 %recovery. Sepsis is number one suspect but it may be difficult to locate a septic focus. Therefore, broad spectrum, third generation cephalosporins may be started empirically. Upper GI bleed, (hematemesis, variceal bleed) is the most common cause. It is postulated that digestion of blood and blood proteins in the gut generates large amount of NH_3 which precipitates HE. Absence of essential aminoacid isoleucine from haemoglobin may make it more aminogenic than other proteins.

Gastric lavage and catharsis are used to clear the gut of the blood. Lactulose 15–20 ml is given orally 2–3 times a day.

Locally acting antibiotics are used. Gut cleansing is the mainstay of management. Hyponatremia if present should be promptly corrected.

3. Concomitant causes should be taken care of.
4. Empirical of HE (Table 5.7)

Lactulose (Fig 5.3). It is a non-absorbable disachharide. The human small intestine does not have enzymes to split these synthetic diasaccharides. They are extensively metabolized by colonic bacteria. The beneficial effect is their ability to reduce the intenstinal production and absorption of ammonia.

Rifaximin. It is a synthetic antibiotic structurally related to rifamycin, has a very low rate of systemic absorption.

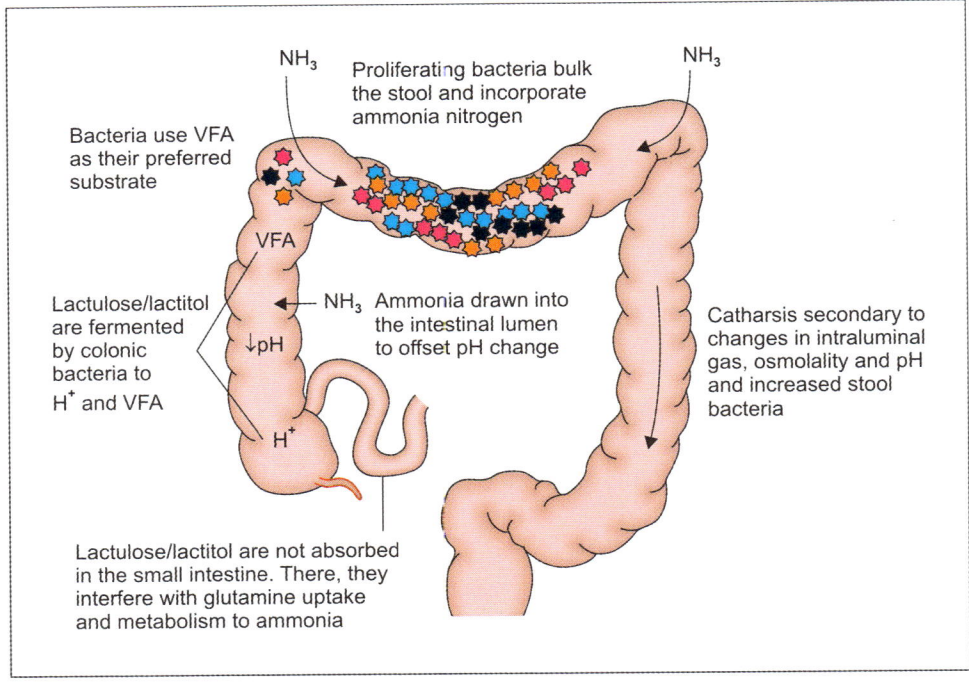

Fig. 5.3: Role of lactulose

Recent US study shows that rifaximin reduces recurrent HE episode in high-risk patients by 58%. It has been suggested that rifaximin is effective in reducing recurrent episodes of HE in patients **where lactulose has failed to do so.**

Other Antibiotics

Neomycin is in use for HE since 1950s. Of late, its toxicity had ended its use. In treatment of HE, antibiotics should have activity against anaerobic bacteria but neomycin does not fit this profile. Recently it has been shown that it inhibits intestinal mucosal enzyme glutaminase which is responsible for production of large amount of ammonia contained in portal vein.

Liver Transplant

When the medical management fails, liver transplantation is required. At present there are many factors to be considered. The most important controversy at present is allocation and distribution of available liver. Various models of end stage liver disease (MELD) have been used.

Effective treatment to prevent or delay the onset of hepatic encephalopathy needs to be developed.

6

Hepatitis

Alaka Deshpande

GENERAL CONSIDERATION

Hepatitis can be defined as an inflammatory liver disease of varied aetiology.

It can be acute, subacute or chronic hepatitis.

AETIOLOGY

- Viral hepatitis
- Enterically transmitted
  - Hepatitis A and hepatitis E
- Parenterally Transmitted
  - Hepatitis B, hepatitis C, and hepatitis D
- Other viruses: Cytomegalovirus (CMV), Herpes simplex virus (HSV), Coxsackie, Epstein-Barr virus (EBV)
- Drug induced hepatitis
- Toxic hepatitis
- Alcohol related hepatitis
- Autoimmune hepatitis

PATHOLOGY

Hepatitis has some common pathological features. It causes an inflammation of the entire liver. The hepatic cell necrosis releases intracellular transaminases. Leukocytic infiltration and histocytic reaction is common. The sinusoids show mononuclear cell infiltration. The reticulin network is usually preserved.

The pathological changes in acute hepatitis of varied aetiology are similar. Therefore, the clinical profile and biochemical features remain similar.

Anorexia, nausea, vomiting, malaise, right hypochondriac pain, high coloured urine are the common symptoms. Depending on the severity of the inflammation, patient may remain anicteric or may go on to develop deep jaundice.

The serum transaminase levels rise. Elevation of aminotransferase more than 10 times the normal is seen in the early stages of inflammation. Elevation of aminotransferase should raise the suspicion of acute hepatitis.

HAV and HEV infection is usually self-limiting. After a variable period the inflammation gradually subsides. The aminotransferase levels return to normal, jaundice may persist for a longer time but gradually disappears. Reticuloendothelial activity increases throughout the recovery phase.

ACUTE VIRAL HEPATITIS

Acute viral hepatitis is a systemic infection though it affects the liver predominantly.

The viral agents causing acute hepatitis are:

Hep A	HAV enterically transmitted
Hep E	HEV enterically transmitted
Hep B	HBV parenterally transmitted
Hep D	HDV parenterally transmitted
Hep C	HCV parenterally transmitted

Transfusion transmitted viruses (TTV) like hepatitis G and others like cytomegalovirus

45

herpes simplex virus, HHV-6, Epstein-Barr virus, HHV-8, can affect liver but do not cause hepatitis.

All the above-mentioned human hepatitis viruses are RNA viruses except HBV which is a DNA virus.

7

Hepatitis A and E

Alaka Deshpande

VIROLOGY

Hepatitis A virus (HAV): It is a RNA virus, 27–28 nm in diameter. It survives exposure to ether, acid environment at pH3. It survived in dried faeces at room temperature for 4 weeks, live oysters for 5 days . It is inactivated at 85°C for 1 minute. The viral taxonomy 1991, classified the virus with new genus hepatovirus.

Hepatitis E virus (HEV): It is a RNA virus, 32–34 nm in diameter classified in a new genus hepevirus. Five major genotypes of HEV have been identified.

Both the infections are transmitted by contaminated water by faeco-oral route. Both are self-limiting infections, however, recent reports have shown HEV as a cause of graft-hepatitis in solid-organ transplant recipients. Although HEV is self-limiting, it is possible that it causes chronic liver disease in some of the immune suppressed individuals.

Pathogenesis

Once HAV is ingested from the contaminated water, it survives the gastric acidity, traverses the mucosa of small intestine and reaches the liver through portal vein. HAV is distributed throughout the liver. It replicates exclusively in hepatocytes. After maturation, it reaches the systemic circulation through hepatic sinusoids and is released through biliary tree, passes into intestine and is excreted in the faeces.

The pathogenesis of hepatic injury is not well-understood. However, the HAV is not a cytopathic virus. Cell damage appears to be immune mediated.

HEV after ingestion reaches the hepatocytes via portal circulation. The pathogenesis of HEV associated liver injury is not completely understood.

Clinical Feature

Clinical features of HAV and HEV infections are similar. In a prodromal stage, the patient complains of malaise, fatigue, increasing anorexia and nausea. Aversion to daily cup of tea, aversion to smoking is classically complained by the patients of hepatitis.

It may be accompanied by vomiting and a high coloured urine. Like other viral infections patients may have arthralgia, myalgia, mild fever and pain in the right hypochondrium. Loss of appetite continues till jaundice appears. As the jaundice becomes apparent the appetite improves and other symptoms gradually subside.

In few cases the icteric phase is followed by cholestasis. 60% of cases show complete clinical recovery in about 2 months. Almost all cases recovers completely in six months.

Hepatitis A may present as:

1. Asymptomatic, without jaundice, diagnosed by raised levels of transaminases.

2. Symptomatic with jaundice, self-limited.
3. Cholestasis with jaundice lasting for about 10 or more weeks.
4. Relapsing with 2 or 3 episodes in 6–10 weeks.
5. Acute liver failure in hyper-endemic region.

Cholestasis. Jaundice deepens and patient starts to itch. Jaundice persists for 2 to 6 months, however the patients feel well. There is no evidence of intra-hepatic dilatation of biliary tree as seen in obstructive jaundice. About 8% of HAV cases and 50% of HEV cases develop cholestasis. The prognosis in usually excellent and clinical recovery is complete.

Acute liver failure is rare in HAV infection. It is reported in less than 2% of cases above the age of 49 years. It manifests in the first week itself and rarely seen after 4 weeks.

It develops rapidly, jaundice deepens in about 7–10 days. Ominous signs are confusion, drowsiness , fetor hepaticus. Haemorrhages may develop. Body temperature rises, jaundice deepens, liver shrinks due to fulminant hepatitis. Fatality rate is high in acute liver failure.

Diagnosis. The diagnosis of hepatitis is based on raised levels of serum transaminases and hyperbilirubinemia.

The incriminating virus is identified by serological detection of specific antiviral antibody, IgM anti-HAV or immunoglobulin M (IgM) anti-HEV. IgM remains positive from the onset of symptoms. Anti-HAV immunoglobulin G (IgG) antibody is also detectable at the onset of the disease and remains present usually for life. Detection of viral RNA is limited to research laboratories at present.

Management. Monitoring of liver function tests at weekly interval is desirable. Transaminase levels start decreasing as the recovery starts. Till then patient is asked to rest. Diet should give adequate calories mainly from carbohydrate diet. There is no basis to avoid fats from the diet as is believed by lay people in India. Antiemetics may be used for nausea-vomiting as required.

Patient should refrain from hepatotoxic agents like paracetamol, nonsteroidal anti-inflammatory drugs (NSAIDs), oral contraceptives, alcohol, etc.

There are no specific antiviral drugs for HAV, HEV, the treatment remains symptomatic.

Prevention. Improved sanitation and prevention of water contamination by sewage is the first pre-requisite. Since the infection spreads by contaminated water, it is necessary to purify the drinking water. Simple boiling of water for 2 minutes kills HAV.

Table 7.1: Enterically transmitted hepatitis		
	HAV	*HEV*
Genome	RNA	RNA
Family	Hepatovirus	Hepevirus
Incubation period	15–45 days	15–60 days
Transmission	Faeco-oral	Faeco-oral
Acute attack	Depends on age	
Anicteric to deep jaundice	Mild	
Diagnosis	Anti-HAV IgM	Anti-HEV IgM
Chronicity	No	Rarely in immunocompromised people
Treatment	Symptomatic	Symptomatic
Prevention	Personal hygiene	Personal hygiene
	Boiled water, milk	Boiled water, milk
	Vaccine	Vaccine (not yet licensed)

Both passive and active immunization is available. Anti-HAV immunoglobulins are given within 2 weeks of exposure in a dose of 0.02 ml/kg.

The HAV vaccine was first licensed in US in 1995. It gives a long-term immunity. For adults above 18 years of age, the dose is 1 ml with a booster dose given 6–12 months later. Immunoglobulins or anti-HEV vaccine is still not available.

In case of acute liver failure due to HEV/HAV, liver transplant may be considered.

8

Hepatitis B and C

Pratibha Sonawane, Deepak Amarapurkar

Hepatitis B viruses (HBV) and hepatitis C virus (HCV), which predominantly transmit through the parenteral route, pose a serious "silent epidemic" challenge to India. Infected persons are unaware of their chronic carrier status, and hence continue to infect others for decades and eventually burden the society with loss of productive workforce, and the health care system with expenses of treating liver failures, chronic liver diseases, and cancers.

Epidemiology of HBV

Worldwide more than two billion people have been infected with hepatitis B virus (HBV) and chronic HBV infection affects about 400 million people. It is estimated that more than 500,000 people die annually due to HBV associated liver disease, largely because of cirrhosis and/or hepatocellular carcinoma. More than 75% of chronically HBV infected patients are in Asia. Despite the availability of safe and effective vaccines for more than two decades, HBV infection is still a global health problem. Economic burden of HBV infection is substantial because of high morbidity and mortality associated with cirrhosis and hepato-cellular carcinoma (HCC).

HBV is the second most common cause of acute viral hepatitis after HEV in India. With 3.7% point prevalence, that is, over 40 million HBV carriers, India is considered to have an intermediate level of HBV endemicity. Every year, one million Indians are at risk for HBV and about 100,000 die from HBV infection.

Virology and Pathogenesis

HBV is a single-stranded DNA virus, with particle size 22 to 42 nano micron with 3.2 kb circular DNA genome. HBV replicates through an RNA intermediate using a virus-encoded reverse transcriptase enzyme. HBV genome has four genes, namely: surface, core, DNA polymerase and X. Four antigens (HBsAg, HBcAg, HBeAg and HB × Ag) have been identified in relation to HBV. Antibodies against this can be detected in the blood and are useful in diagnosis of various phases of HBV infection. There are at least 7 HBV genotypes (from A to G). Genotype D and A are more common in India. In immuno-competent persons, HBV is not cytopathic, and liver damage in this infection is caused through an immune-mediated mechanism directed against HBV-infected hepatocytes. However, in post-transplant patients, the virus appears to produce liver damage via a cytopathic effect.

Modes of Transmission

HBV is transmitted by blood-borne route, such as transfusion of infected blood and blood products, intravenous drug use, haemodialysis, sexual contact, percutaneous exposure (like needle-stick injuries, shared razor blades and tooth brushes, tattooing, acupuncture, etc.), and mother-to-newborn (i.e. perinatal) transmission. In India, a majority of chronic HBV infections are acquired horizontally, and less than 20% of chronic HBV infections results from vertical mother-to-child transmission.

Natural History

The incubation period for HBV is 60 days, and it can vary from 28 to 160 days. Approximately 30% of infections among adults present as icteric hepatitis, and 0.1–0.5% of patients develop fulminant hepatitis. Almost 25% of persons who acquire infection in neonatal stages develop complications like cirrhosis, decompensation and hepatocellular carcinoma. HBV infection leads to one of four outcomes:

- Recovery after acute infection (>95% in previously healthy adults over the age of 40).
- Fulminant hepatitis
- Chronic hepatitis B (can progress to cirrhosis and hepatocellular carcinoma)
- Inactive carrier state

The outcome of HBV infection depends on immunological factors and possibly in part on the characteristics of the virus. The age at which the infection occurs plays a very important role. When it is acquired perinatally and in infants under 1 year of age, chronic infection will develop in 80–90% of cases; in children between the ages of 1 and 5, 30–50% will go on to develop chronic infection. By comparison, 30–50% of adults who become actively infected with HBV are symptomatic, but only 2–6% of these adults develop chronic infection. Some 95–99% of previously healthy adults with an acute HBV infection recover completely. In chronically infected persons, 70 to 90% are asymptomatic chronic carrier whereas only 10 to 30% develop chronic hepatitis. 30% of chronic hepatitis B persons progresses to liver cirrhosis with further decompensation is seen in 4% patients per year. Hepatocellular carcinoma developes at the rate of 2–8% per year in liver cirrhosis

patients and 0.1% per year in chronic carriers. Chronic hepatitis B infection evolves in 4 different phases:

1. Immune tolerant,
2. Immune clearance,
3. Residual- nonreplicative, and
4. Reactivation.

1. *Immune tolerant phase.* HBsAg and HBeAg are detectable, HBV DNA levels are high, but aminotransferase are normal or minimally elevated and mostly asymptomatic. It is during the replication of virus that liver suffers injury; usually it lasts for 20–30 years with very low spontaneous HBsAg clearance rate of 2–3% per year and annual risk for HCC 0.5%.

2. *Immune clearance phase.* During second or third decades of chronic infection, HBV DNA levels decrease and aminotransferase levels increase, patient becomes symptomatic and experiences flares of aminotransferase. In some this is followed by HBeAg seroconversion and very low HBV DNA levels that are suppressed by host immunity reasonably, this evolve as inactive carriers or may lead to resolution of HBV infection with spontaneous HBeAg clearance rate up to 10–20% per year. In some (1–5%), seroconversion is accompanied by selection of HBV mutants and results in HBeAg negative hepatitis B.

3. *Residual phase.* Inactive carrier stage with HBeAg negativity, antiHBe positivity, undetectable HBV DNA and normal alanine aminotransferase (ALT). Histology depends on duration of disease prior to seroconversion.

In adults hepatitis B infection consists of two phases; an earlier replicative phase with active disease and non-replicative phase with remission of liver disease. In neonates there is first phase of immunotolerance during which virus replicates actively without liver disease, followed by second phase of immune clearance where patients develop hepatitis with clearance of virus replication and the third phase low replication persists during which mutants may develop.

4. *Reactivation:* In some, liver disease may relapse after period of inactivity.

Clinical Features

Spectrum of symptomatology of hepatitis B is very wide. Anicteric hepatitis is the predominant form of expression of this disease. The majority of the patients are asymptomatic, but patients with anicteric hepatitis have a greater tendency to develop chronic hepatitis. Patients with symptomatology have the same symptoms as patients who develop icteric hepatitis. Icteric hepatitis is associated with a prodromal period, during which a serum sickness-like syndrome can occur. The symptomatology is more constitutional and includes anorexia, nausea, vomiting, low-grade fever, myalgia, fatigability, disordered gustatory acuity and smell sensations (aversion to foods). Also, right upper quadrant and epigastric pain (intermittent, mild to moderate) is common.

Patients with fulminant and subfulminant hepatitis may present with hepatic encephalopathy in the form of somnolence, disturbances in sleep pattern, mental confusion and coma. Patients can also present with ascites, gastrointestinal (GI) bleeding and coagulopathy.

Patients with chronic hepatitis B disease can be immune tolerant or have an inactive chronic infection without any evidence of active disease; they are also asymptomatic. Patients with chronic active hepatitis, especially during the replicative state, may complain of symptoms similar to those of acute hepatitis.

If progressive liver disease is present, then hepatic decompensation in the form of hepatic encephalopathy, ascites, GI bleeding and coagulopathy can occur.

Extraepatic manifestations include arthralgia, polyarteritis nodosa, pericarditis, thrombocytopenia, glomerulonephritis, pancreatitis, aplastic anaemia and mixed essential cryoglobulinaemia.

Laboratory Investigations

Laboratory evaluation for hepatitis B disease generally consists of liver enzyme tests, including levels of alanine aminotransferase (ALT) and/or aspartate aminotransferase (AST), alkaline phosphatase (ALP), and gamma-glutamyl transpeptidase (GGT), as well as liver function tests (LFTs) that include total and direct serum bilirubin, albumin, and measurement of the international normalized ratio (INR). Hematologic and coagulation studies also include a platelet count and a complete blood count (CBC).

To evaluate the patient's level of infectivity, quantification of HBV DNA is essential, and the presence of hepatitis B e antigen (HBeAg) should be determined. Indeed, the best indication of active viral replication is the presence of HBV DNA in the serum. Hybridization or more sensitive polymerase chain reaction (PCR) assay techniques are used to detect the viral genome in the serum, as well as specific genotypes, mutants resistant to oral nucleoside and nucleotide analogues, and core and precore mutations. But these investigations are not required routinely. HBV DNA testing is also recommended when occult HBV is suspected (positive anti-HBc and negative antibody to hepatitis B surface antigen [anti-HBs] and hepatitis B surface antigen [HBsAg]) or in cases in which all of the serologic tests are negative.

Diagnosis of HBV infection is based on estimating various antigens and antibodies in the sera while demonstration of HBV DNA in the sera of liver tissue. Presence of HBsAg (i.e. Australia antigen) in the blood suggests that patient is infected with HBV. Presence of HBeAg in the blood suggests active viral replication. IgM anti-HBC antibodies indicate acute infection. Anti-HBc IgG antibodies remain in the blood lifelong after exposure to HBV. Anti-HBs antibodies development with disappearance of HBsAg suggest complete recovery from HBV infection. Assessing HBV DNA by polymerase chain reaction is useful tool in judging the response to treatment and estimating mutant viruses.

Treatment of Hepatitis B Infection

Acute HBV infection in majority of adults is a self-limiting disease and hence does not require any antiviral treatment. In addition, appropriate measures should be taken to prevent infection in exposed contacts. Careful follow-up of these patients especially in children is required to catch those patients who are going to develop chronicity.

The approach to the treatment of chronic HBV infection has dramatically changed over the past decade and the current availability of a number of antiviral drugs adds to the complexity of management of chronic HBV. Current treatments for hepatitis B are very effective at controlling or suppressing the hepatitis B virus. However, hepatitis B treatment only rarely leads to "cure".

Drugs available for treatment of hepatitis B: There are two classes of drugs used in the treatment of HBV 1. immunomodulators, 2. oral antiviral agents. Interferon and peginterferon are the immunomodulators licensed for treatment of HBV. No drug resistance has been reported with the use of these agents. All these agents are injectable, expensive, with significant side-effects and have limited efficacy.

Oral antiviral agents for treatment of HBV are lamivudine, adefovir, entecavir, telbivudine and tenofovir. Currently, pegylated interferon alfa (PEG-IFN-α), entecavir (ETV), and tenofovir disoproxil fumarate (TDF) are the first-line agents in the treatment of hepatitis B. These are the main treatment drugs approved globally for this. Emtricitabine and tenofovir are available for treatment of HBV and HIV co-infections. Lamivudine (3TC),

telbivudine, and adefovir are currently considered second or third-line therapy, or "non-preferred" treatment.

Long-term use of oral antiviral agents can effectively suppress hepatitis B virus DNA, leading to decrease in incidence of hepatitic flares, as well as in the development of cirrhosis and hepatocellular carcinoma. Still the presence of intracellular covalently closed circular DNA (cccDNA) in hepatocytes cannot be eliminated with the current therapies. Cure of HBV infection remains elusive. Treatment end point of disappearance of surface antigen can be achieved only in minority patients. Hence treatment practically needs to be continued lifelong. Efficacy and safety data of these agents beyond 5 years is not yet available.

Goals of Treatment for Chronic HBV Infection

Active HBV replication is the key driver of liver injury and disease progression. Therefore, the primary aim of chronic hepatitis B treatment is to permanently suppress HBV replication. Clinically, the short-term goal of treatment is to achieve 'initial response' in terms of HBeAg seroconversion and/or HBV-DNA suppression, ALT normalization, and prevention of hepatic decompensation, and to ensure 'maintained/sustained response' to reduce hepatic necroinflammation and fibrosis during/after therapy. The ultimate long-term goal of therapy is to prevent hepatic decompensation, reduce or prevent progression to cirrhosis and/or HCC, and prolong survival.

Over last two decades several guidelines by various associations have been published and updated from time to time. The treatment indications in these guidelines are based on HBV DNA levels, SGPT levels, HBeAg status and presence of fibrosis and cirrhosis. Limitations of current practice guidelines are:

1. Our knowledge about the natural history of HBV infection is still evolving,
2. Normal level of SGPT is a matter of great controversy,

3. Cut-off limits of HBV DNA for starting treatment are not clear,

4. Treatment endpoints especially in HBeAg negative patients are not well-defined, treatment strategies for primary treatment failure or previously drug exposed patients is not yet clear. Indication for treatment as per these guidelines is summarized in the Table 8.7.

Treatment of patients with cirrhosis should not be based on ALT levels, as these may be normal in advanced disease. Interferon alpha increases the risk of sepsis and decompensation in patients with advanced cirrhosis. However, interferon can be used for the treatment of well-compensated cirrhosis. The use of potent nucleoside analogues with very low-risk of resistance, i.e. tenofovir or entecavir, is particularly relevant in this group of patients. Close monitoring of HBV DNA levels is important and resistance must be prevented by adding a second drug without cross-resistance if HBV DNA is not undetectable at week 48 of therapy. If lamivudine has to be prescribed (because of local policy), it should be used in combination with adefovir or preferably tenofovir. Thus patients with cirrhosis require long-term therapy, with careful monitoring for resistance and flares. Clinical studies indicate that prolonged and adequate suppression of HBV DNA may stabilize patients and delay or even obviate need for transplantation. Partial regression of fibrosis has been reported.

Treatment of patients with decompensated cirrhosis: Patients with decompensated cirrhosis should be treated in specialized liver units, as the application of antiviral therapy is complex, and these patients may be candidates for liver transplantation. End-stage liver disease should be treated as a matter of urgency. Treatment is indicated even if HBV DNA level is low in order to prevent recurrent reactivation. Potent nucleoside analogues with good resistance profiles (entecavir or tenofovir) should be used. However, there are little data for the safety of these agents in decompensated cirrhosis. Patients may show slow clinical improvement over a period of 3–6 months. However, some patients with advanced hepatic disease with a high Child-Pugh or MELD score may have progressed beyond the point of no return, and may not benefit, thus requiring transplantation if possible. In that situation, treatment with NUCs will decrease the risk of HBV recurrence in the graft.

Treatment of patients with acute liver failure: Should be treated with oral antivirals.

Prevention of HBV Infection

HBV infection can be prevented by screening blood for HBsAg, using disposable needles and syringes, using gloves and practicing safe sex. Both active and passive immunization are available. Genetically engineered recombinant vaccines as well as plasma-derived vaccines have more than 95% efficacy and high safety profile. Hepatitis B immunoglobulin is useful in post-exposure prophylaxis (i.e. within 48 hours) and prevents maternofetal transmission of HBV. Vaccination can be effectively used to reduce HBV infection rate and to reduce the incidence of hepatocellular carcinoma. HBV vaccination should be integrated into expanded programme of immunization in all children. Various vaccination schedules like 0, 1, 6 months or 0, 1, 2, and 12 months are equally effective. After successful vaccination booster dose is not required for at least 20 years. India introduced universal immunization against hepatitis B in 10 states in the year 2002, and in 2011, scaled up this operation countrywide. Recently a pentavalent vaccine, which also protects against HBV, has been introduced in some states. The HBV vaccine also protects from HDV infection.

Recommendations for Hepatitis B Vaccinations

- Routine immunization
  - All infants and previously unvaccinated children (by age 2 year)

- Increased risk
  - People with multiple sexual partners.
  - Household contacts and sexual partners of HBV carriers.
  - Men having sex with men
  - Injection drug users
  - Persons travelling to or working in countries with high or intermediate rates of disease.
  - Individuals with occupational risk of disease (e.g. health care workers).
  - Clients/staff or institutions for developmentally disabled.
  - Patients with chronic renal failure.
  - Hematologic conditions requiring multiple transfusions and recipients of clotting factor concentrates.

Screening for Chronic Hepatitis B

More than two-thirds of patients are unaware of their infection and less than half of the patients who are diagnosed to have chronic HBV infection are referred to specialist for further evaluation and management. Screening should be done in:

- All pregnant women.
- All chronic hemodialysis patients.
- HIV-positive people.
- People with unexplained abnormal liver enzyme levels.
- Children born to hepatitis B-infected mothers after completion of the vaccine series.
- All foreign born people (including immigrants and internationally adopted children) from geographic areas with chronic hepatitis B virus prevalence of 2% or greater, including Asia, the Pacific Islands, Africa, and Eastern Europe.
- All unvaccinated US born people with at least one foreign-born parent from geographic areas with chronic hepatitis B virus prevalence of 2% or greater, including Asia, the Pacific Islands, Africa, and Eastern Europe.

Tests to be performed depend on the purpose of the screening.

- *Hepatitis B surface antigen:* presence indicates active infection, further evaluation is indicated.
- *Hepatitis B surface antibody:* presence indicates immunity, vaccination is not necessary.
- *Hepatitis B core antibody (total):* presence indicates prior or ongoing infection, further evaluation is necessary to differentiate whether infection is ongoing (hepatitis B surface antigen-positive) or resolved (hepatitis B surface antibody-positive).

Summary: Tests for Determining Treatment Candidacy for HBV

- Determining treatment candidacy at its most basic is a simple 2-step process of measuring
  - HBV DNA
  - ALT
- However, often important to consider other parameters to individualize treatment
  - HBV DNA and ALT assessment
  - Family history of HCC
  - Coinfection assessment
  - Precore, core, and genotype
  - Alcohol or metabolic syndrome
  - Liver biopsy or advanced imaging for fibrosis
  - AFP

Hepatitis C (HCV)

Over the past few years, HCV treatment has witnessed a paradigm shift. With the advent of newer directly acting antiviral agents, high cure rates have been obtained in favourable genotypes. What was once considered a chronic non-curable disease, can now be completely eradicated. Though, the initial treatment results have been generally favourable, long-term follow-up is the need of the hour to comment upon the safety and efficacy of the new treatment regimens.

Hepatitis C virus (HCV) was discovered in the late 1980s, when it was learned that most non-A, non-B hepatitis were infected with HCV. It has been demonstrated that 20%–30% of patients infected with HCV progress to cirrhosis over a span of 20–30 years and a fraction from these can progress to hepatocellular carcinoma (HCC). HCV, at present, is one of the leading causes for liver transplantation in the west. Certainly, modern hepatology has had the most important discovery in terms of research in the virology, epidemiology, and therapeutics regarding HCV.

HCV

HCV is a single stranded positive sense enveloped RNA virus of 50 nm in diameter and belongs to Flaviviridae family and *Hepacivirus* genus. Hepatocytes are the major site of viral replication, although viral replication also occurs in blood mononuclear cells, B-cells, T-cells and dendritic cells. HCV shows considerable heterogeneity throughout the genome due to an inherently high mutational rate. Some mutations are lethal to virus whereas some gives advantage to virus by evading or inhibiting host immune response. Viral genotype is a genetically distinct group of HCV isolates which arises during evolution of the virus. There are 6 genotype and more than 70 subtypes of HCV. HCV genotype does not influence the severity of liver disease but it correlate well with treatment response. HCV genotype does not change over time and hence need to be done only once in an infected person. Distribution of HCV genotypes shows global geographic differences. In India, genotype 3 is reported to be the most prevalent, followed by genotype 1.

Epidemiology

Prevalence

The most recent estimates published in 2004 indicated that 2.2%, or 120 to 130 million people, are infected with HCV worldwide. However, as the prevalence data is patchy and incomplete from many areas of the world, the true prevalence is underestimated. The World Health Organization reports the highest estimated prevalence of HCV infection in Africa (5.3%) followed by the eastern Mediterranean region (4.6%), western Pacific region (3.9%), Southeast Asia (2.2%), and Europe (1%). The prevalence of HCV infection in southern European countries such as Spain, Italy, and Greece ranges between 2.5% and 3.5%, compared to a prevalence of <1% in northern European regions such as the United Kingdom and Scandinavia. Similarly, one of the highest rates of HCV infection is noted in Egypt where the prevalence is estimated at 11–14%.

The World Health Organization estimates that there are 10–24 million HCV-infected persons living in India. Estimates of the prevalence of HCV infection in India vary from <1% among voluntary blood donors to >90% among injection drug users (IDUs). There is no national surveillance system in India, and presently the epidemiology is described by isolated studies and blood bank data. The estimated HCV prevalence has been 1–1.9% in India.

Incidence

Since 1989, United States has witnessed a decline in the number of estimated new infections by more than 80% to fewer than 30,000 estimated new infections per year. With the screening of blood for the virus with anti-HCV testing and, more lately, nucleic acid testing (NAT), as well as education in IDU populations, the incidence is definitely reducing. However, the morbidity and mortality related to chronic hepatitis C and its complications continue to rise, especially in developing countries as a result of delay in diagnosis.

Risk Factors and Modes of Transmission

Several risk factors account for the majority of cases of transmission of hepatitis C, including intravenous drug use, blood transfusions from unscreened donors, and iatrogenic exposure from unsafe injection practices. In developed countries such as the United States, the European continent, and Australia, intravenous drug use is the most common risk factor for acquiring hepatitis C. Among long-term injection drug users the prevalence of hepatitis C infection has been reported to be as high as 94%. Although sharing syringes has been most frequently implicated in the transmission of HCV, the shared use of other drug preparation equipment may have contributed to infection in an estimated 37% of recent HCV infections.

In developing countries like India, unsafe therapeutic injection practices, where syringes or needles may be reused without sterilization, continues to contribute to incident cases of hepatitis C and remains a major transmission risk for blood-borne infections. Patients who received blood transfusions prior to 1992 are considered to be at risk for hepatitis C infection with an odds ratio of 2.6 compared with individuals who did not receive transfusions, and older patients are more likely to have acquired HCV infection as a result of blood transfusions. In India, mandatory screening for HCV was introduced as late as 2002. Overall, it has been estimated that past blood transfusions account for about 10% of cases of chronic hepatitis C. Certain population of patients requiring multiple transfusions are at extraordinary risk for hepatitis C infection, like thalassemia and hemophilia. The sexual transmission is extremely rare and usually occurs only under special circumstances. The presence of HIV infection, on the other hand, has regularly been associated with a higher likelihood of sexual transmission of HCV in both heterosexuals and among men who have sex with men (MSM). The perinatal transmission rate from HCV RNA-positive mothers is estimated to range between 4% and 10%. The rate increases substantially to between 6% and 23% when the mother is co-infected with HIV. An increased risk of perinatal transmission appears to be associated with higher levels of maternal HCV RNA. Recent recommendations by the Centre for Disease Control established that for women with chronic hepatitis C infection who are uninfected with HIV, no changes to routine delivery and breastfeeding are required. However, for mothers co-infected with HCV and HIV, elective caesarean delivery with no breastfeeding (when safe infant formula is available) are recommended in order to diminish the risk of neonatal transmission. Obstetric procedures such as amniocentesis and invasive monitoring with foetal scalp electrodes have been associated with an increased risk of neonatal transmission.

The likelihood of acquiring hepatitis C from a needle-stick injury from an HCV-infected patient is estimated to be approximately 2%. Rare cases of blood splash exposure have been reported. A larger inoculum is associated with a higher risk of transmission, injuries with hollow bore needles transmit HCV more frequently than solid instruments. Similarly, higher levels of viremia, higher is the risk of transmission. Health care workers who sustain a needle-stick injury from an index case with hepatitis C should be reassured about the low rate of infection. There is no role for postexposure prophylaxis. Baseline liver enzymes and anti-HCV antibody should be obtained immediately and follow-up testing performed at 1, 3, and 6 months. Patients with evidence of acute infection should be followed to determine if spontaneous resolution will occur or be treated within 12–16 weeks after infection in order to maximize the chances of cure.

Patients with end-stage renal disease (ESRD) on maintenance hemodialysis (MHD) are at increased risk for acquiring HCV infection as a result of cross-contamination from the dialysis circuits. In addition, these patients are often anaemic and require multiple blood transfusions. Because of the variety of human activities that involve the potential for percutaneous exposure to blood or blood-derived body fluids, there are numerous other biologically plausible modes of transmission besides those with clearly demonstrated epidemiologic associations with infection. These include cosmetic procedures (tattooing, body piercing), intranasal drug use, and religious or cultural practices such as ritual scarification, circumcision and acupuncture.

Pathogenesis

The pathogenesis of HCV infection is quite complex and regulated by viral factors as well as host factors. Whereas both innate and adaptive immunity are involved in the pathogenic action of HCV, the CD8+ cytotoxic lymphocytes are crucial in deciding the eradication or persistence of viral particles. HCV is not cytopathic. The host's immune response leading to long-lasting inflammation in an attempt to fight the virus is the cause of liver damage. Acute self-limiting HCV infection is associated with a strong and consistent multi-specific CD4+ and CD8+ T-cell responses against the epitopes of viral proteins. The probable reasons for the persistence of HCV despite such responses are:

1. Extensive mutations during HCV replication, leading to multiple viral species in a single patient known as quacispecies;
2. Mutations that prevent antigen presentation;
3. The inhibition of intracellular interferon (IFN) signalling;
4. The functional impairment of natural killer cell and CD8+ T-lymphocyte responses; and
5. Viral inhibition of host defences.

Natural History of HCV Infection

Patients with acute hepatitis C are usually asymptomatic or subclinical. It accounts for about 20% of cases of acute hepatitis. Most studies have reported high (70–85%) rates of progression from acute to chronic hepatitis C, but the transition from acute disease to cirrhosis is usually symptom-free, and occurs over a period of 20–40 years in approximately 5–25% of HCV infected patients. Hepatocellular carcinoma may develop in as many as 1–4% of patients with established cirrhosis per year. The main pathway of cirrhosis development is progressive liver fibrosis, the stage of which is the main prognostic factor in the natural history of chronic hepatitis C. Patients with persistently high aminotransferase levels and necro-inflammatory activity at liver biopsy are likely to develop more fibrosis. The progression of fibrosis is faster in males and in Afro-Americans, as well as in subjects consuming large amounts of alcohol, diabetics, and those with pathological lipid metabolism, HIV and HBV co-infections or other co-factors.

Clinical Features

Most patients with acute and chronic hepatitis C infection are asymptomatic or may have non-specific symptoms such as fatigue or malaise. Symptoms characteristic of complications from advanced or decompensated liver disease are often related to portal hypertension which includes mental status changes (hepatic encephalopathy), ankle oedema and abdominal distention (ascites), and hematemesis or malena (variceal bleeding).

Symptoms may first develop as clinical findings of extrahepatic manifestations of HCV and most commonly involve the joints, muscle, and skin. About 40–70% of HCV patients develop at least one extra-hepatic manifestation (EHM) and, as many patients do not show any hepatic symptoms of chronic HCV infection, EHMs may be the first signs of the disease. The most commonly occurring extra-hepatic manifestations are as follows:

- Arthralgias
- Membranoproliferative glomerulonephritis
- Idiopathic thrombocytopenic purpura
- Lichen planus
- Paresthesias
- Myalgias
- Mixed cryoglobulinaemia
- Non-Hodgkin lymphoma
- Autoimmune thyroiditis
- Sicca syndrome

In addition, sensory neuropathy has been reported as an extra-hepatic manifestation in patients with HCV infection. Patients also present with symptoms that are less specific and are often unaccompanied by discrete dermatologic findings. Pruritus and urticaria are examples of less specific clues to underlying HCV infection in the appropriate setting (e.g. post-transfusion, organ transplantation, surgery, intravenous drug use).

Laboratory investigations

Serological testing for anti-HCV antibody is most commonly used method for screening. Testing is usually done using enzyme immune assay (EIA). But it could not differentiate between acute, chronic and resolved infection. Anti-HCV EIAs include second and third generation EIAs. These assays are 97% specific. The most recent third-generation EIA detects antibodies against core protein and non-structural proteins 3, 4, and 5 and can yield positive results an average of 8 weeks after the onset of infection.

False-negative results for the presence of HCV antibody can occur in persons with immune compromised status like those with HIV, chronic kidney disease, HCV-associated essential mixed cryoglobulinemia and patients on dialysis. False-positive EIA results can also occur. The likelihood of a false-positive result is greater in persons without risk factors and in those without signs of liver disease, such as blood donors or health care workers.

Quantitative or qualitative HCV RNA assay is commonly used to confirm the diagnosis. Qualitative assays detect HCV RNA in blood using amplification techniques such as PCR or transcription-mediated amplification (TMA). Quantitative assays ascertain HCV RNA quantity in blood, using target amplification techniques (PCR, TMA) or signal amplification (branched DNA [bDNA] assay). The change in HCV RNA level can also be used to monitor treatment response.

Once the diagnosis is confirmed, baseline studies like complete blood cell count (CBC) with differential, liver function tests, including alanine aminotransferase (ALT) level and thyroid function tests should be done. HCV genotyping has to done once as an aid for guiding treatment. Screening tests for coinfection with HIV or hepatitis B virus (HBV) are necessary. Non-invasive test for liver fibrosis like fibroscan and ARFI scan can be used to assess degree of liver fibrosis although liver biopsy remains gold standard.

Treatment

Antiviral therapy should be considered in all patients with chronic hepatitis C. Goal of HCV treatment is to achieve sustained eradication of HCV RNA and prevent progression to cirrhosis, hepatocellular carcinoma and decompensated liver disease. Treatment responses are defined as:

Biochemical response: Normalization of serum ALT level.

Virological response: Undetectable serum HCV RNA by PCR.

Histological response: > 2-point improvement in necro-inflammatory score with no worsening in fibrosis score

Treatment duration is decided based on presence or absence of cirrhosis, HCV genotype and previous treatment exposure. The treatment of hepatitis C has evolved over the years. Initial studies used IFN monotherapy followed by combination of ribavirin and IFN. Later, IFN was switched to pegalyted INF (INF to which polyethylene glycol (PEG) molecules have been added, i.e. PEG-IFN). Protease inhibitors have emerged as a third feature of combination therapy. The first protease inhibitor indicated for use in HCV infection, boceprevir, was approved by the FDA in May 2011 followed by approval of telaprevir. However, these two protease inhibitors are not recommended due to the more recent availability of more effective options. A third protease inhibitor, simeprevir was approved in November 2013 and is recommended as a part of combination therapy for chronic hepatitis C infection. More recently, HCV NS5B polymerase inhibitor sofosbuvir (Sovaldi) was shown to result in suppression of HCV replication and has emerged as an important component of currently recommended regimens. Currently among directly acting antiviral, sofosbuvir is available in India. Specific considerations are needed for persons with HIV/HCV coinfection, decompensated cirrhosis, post-liver transplant HCV infection, and those with severe renal impairment or end-stage renal disease (ESRD). They should be managed by specialist.

Until 2011, the historically accepted standard therapy with pegylated interferon and ribavirin produced an SVR rate of approximately 40–50% for genotype 1 patients and higher rates up to 80% for alternate genotypes after 24–48 weeks of therapy. In addition interferon and ribavirin has many side-effects. Ribavarin is contraindicated in pregnant patients or those with advanced renal disease. Likewise, interferon therapy is contraindicated in patients with autoimmune diseases, uncontrolled depression and mental illness, decompensated liver disease or decompensated cardiac or pulmonary disease.

Newer therapies directed against specific viral and host targets appear to have greater potential for success.

Sofosbuvir based regimes have improved SVR rate to 80% to 90% in treatment naive and non-cirrhotic population. In cirrhotic patients SVR of 50% to 60% can be achieved using these combinations. Overall advanced cirrhosis patients shows poor response rate and often do not tolerate complete treatment. Interferon free regimes are approved for treatment of HCV but all the drugs are still not available in India. Only available directly acting antiviral in India is sofosbuvir. Ledipasvir will be soon available in near future. Sofosbuvir is very safe drug and devoid of any major drug-drug interaction. Also it is effective against all genotype. Monotherapy with directly acting antiviral is to be strictly avoided as it carries risk of future resistance. The summary of recent AASLD recommendation for treatment for HCV is given in Table 8.1 to 8.10.

Table 8.1: Hepatitis B and "C" in nut shell		
	Hepatitis B	Hepatitis C
Years after discovery	50 years	25 years
Virus	42 nm DNA virus (Hepadnavirus Family)	50 nm RNA virus (Flaviviridae Family)
Antigen	Surface antigen of HBsAg	HCV antigens (assays not commercially available)
Antibodies	Anti-HBc IgM (acute, rarely chronic), and anti-HBc IgG (acute, chronic or convalescent Anti HBS (neutrallizing, seen post-recovery or after vaccination; rarely chronic)	Anti HCV
Epidemiology in India	1–3%	0.2–1%
Chronicity in adults	2–10%	85–95%
Prevention	Pre-exposure: Active hepatitis B Vaccine	No vaccine
	Post-exposure—hepatitis B Immunoglobulin	Globulin unavailable; avoid high-risk behaviours
Mortality in general population	0.01	0.01
Mortality in pregnant women	0.01	0.01
Risk of perinatal transmission	3+	3+
Curative treatment	Not available	Available

Table 8.2: Who should be screened?

Hepatitis B	Hepatitis C
1. Infants born to infected mothers	1. Recipients of clotting factor concentrates before 1987
2. Sex partners of infected persons	2. Recipients of blood transfusions or donated organs before universal screening for hepatitis C started
3. Persons with multiple sex partners	3. Long-term hemodialysis patients
4. Persons with a sexually transmitted disease (STD) men who have sex with men	4. Health care workers after needlesticks injury
5. Household contacts of infected persons	5. HIV-infected persons
6. Health care and public safety workers exposed to blood on the job	6. Infants born to infected mothers
7. Hemodialysis patients	7. Recipients of blood or organs from a donor who later tested positive for HCV
8. Residents and staff of facilities for developmentally disabled persons	
9. Travelers to regions with intermediate or high rates of hepatitis B (HBsAg prevalence of >2%)	

Table 8.3: Transmission of HBV and HCV infection

	HBV	HCV
Mother to baby	4+	1+
Transfusion (blood, blood products)	4+	4+
Fluids (blood, semen)	4+	2+
Organs and tissue transplantation	4+	4+
Contaminated needle and syringes	4+	4+
Child to child	4+	1+

Table 8.4: Risk of transmission of hepatitis B and C HIV infection by needlestick injuries

Virus	Risk of transmission
Hepatitis B	10 to 30%
Hepatitis C	0.5 to 1%
HIV	0.1 to 0.5%

Table 8.5: Definitions

HBV infection	Presence of HBsAg/HBVDNA in serum/liver
Acute hepatitis B	History, raised ALT, HBsAg +ve and IgM antiHBc +ve
Chronic hepatitis B with active liver disease	Chronic necro-inflammation Diagnostic criteria-HBsAg +ve > 6 months, HBV DNA more than 10^5 copies/ml, elevated ALT/AST and liver biopsy-necroinflammatory score > 4
Inactive HBsAg carrier state	Persistent HBV infection without necroinflammation Diagnostic criteria—HBsAg +ve > 6 months, no sign/symptoms, normal AST and ALT, HBeAg –ve, Anti-HBe +ve, HBVDNA < 10^5 copies/ml, liver biopsy-necroinflammatory score <4
Resolved hepatitis B	Previous HBV infection without active viral infection presently Diagnostic criteria—history of acute or chronic hepatitis B or presence of Anti-HBc + Anti-HBs, HBsAg –ve, undetectable HBVDNA and normal ALT
Occult HBV	Undetectable HBsAg but HBVDNA +ve in serum or liver

Table 8.6: Various drugs available for treatment of chronic hepatitis B

Drug	Mode of administration	Dosage	Duration	Response of resistance	Development of resistance	Safety	Cost of therapy Indian	Cost therapy international brand
Interferon	S.C.	6 MIU daily	24 wk	30–40%	No	Poor	57,000 ($ 1000)	144,000 ($2,500)
Peginterferon interferon	S.C.	1.5 mg/kg body wt weekly	48 wk	40–45%	No	Poor	385,000 ($ 6,800)	816,000 ($14,500)
Thymosin alpha	S.C.	1.6 mg S.C. twice a week	48 wk	30–40%	No	Good	70,000 ($1,300)	800,000 ($ 14,000)
Lamivudine	Oral	100 mg	> 48 wk	18%	20–80% from 1 to 4 years	Excellent	2,400 ($42)	7,200 ($126)
Adefovir	Oral	10 mg	> 48 wk	12%	0–20% from 1–4 years	Excellent	7,200 ($ 126)	95,000 ($1642)
Entacavir	Oral	0.5 or 1 mg	> 48 wk	30%	No resistance to naïve patients for 2 years 5–12% in 2 years in LAM treated patients	Excellent	24,000 ($ 420)	70,000 ($1,230)
Telbuvidine	Oral	600 mg	> 48 wk	20%	4–12% in two years	Excellent	18,000 ($ 316)	60,000 ($1,052)
Tenovofir	Oral	300 mg	> 48 wk	30%	0%- up 5 to 3 yrs	Excellent	16,200 ($285)	30,000 ($ 525)

Table 8.7: Treatment recommendations for chronic hepatitis B

	HBeAg positive patients		HBeAg negative patients	
	APASL 2012	EASL 2012	APASL 2012	EASL 2012
Whom to treat	ALT > 2 upper limit of normal HBV DNA > 2 × 10^4 IU/mL	ALT > upper limit of normal HBV DNA > 2 × 10^3 IU/mL	ALT > 2 upper limit of normal HBV DNA > 2 × 10^3 IU/mL	ALT > upper limit of normal HBV DNA > 2 × 10^3 IU/mL
	Any ALT and HBV DNA +ve in cirrhosis	Any ALT and HBV DNA +ve in cirrhosis	Any ALT and HBV DNA +ve in cirrhosis	Any ALT and HBV DNA +ve in cirrhosis
Preferred drugs	Interferon, peg interferon, ETV, TDF, ADV, LDT and LAM	Peg interferon, ETV, TDF	Interferon, peg interferon, ETV, TDF, ADV, LDT and LAM	Peg interferon, ETV, TDF
Duration of treatment	Peg INF-48 weeks	Peg INF-48 weeks	Peg INF-48 weeks	Peg INF-48 weeks
	For NUCs-1 yr after e-seroconversion	For NUCs-till clearance for HBsAg	For NUCs-till HBsAg-ve or HBV DNA-ve on 3 separate occasions 6 months apart	For NUCs-till clearance for HBsAg

Table 8.8: Treatment response definition: Aim is to achieve SVR

Rapid virological response RVR	**Undetectable HCV RNA in a sensitive assay at week 4 of therapy**
Early virological response EVR	HCV RNA detectable at week 4 but undetectable at week 12, maintained up to end of treatment
Sustained virological response	Undetectable HCV RNA in a sensitive assay at week 12–24 week of completion of therapy
Delayed virological response DVR	More than 2 log10 IU/ml decrease from baseline but detectable HCV RNA at week 12, then undetectable at 24 wk and maintained up to end of treatment
Null response NR	Less than 2 log10 IU/ml decrease in HCV RNA level from baseline at 12 wk of therapy
Partial response PR	More than 2 log10 IU/ml decrease in HCV RNA level from baseline at 12 wk of therapy but HCV RNA detectable at 24 wk
Breakthrough BT	Reappearance of HCV RNA at anytime during treatment after a negative result or increase of 1 log10 IU/ml from nadir

Table 8.9: Commonly used drugs for HCV

Drug	Dose
Pegylated interferon alfa-2a	180 ug per week
Pegylated interferon alfa-2b	1.5ug/kg per week
Ribavirin	For IFN based regime: Genotype 1 and 4–13.3 mg/kg/day in two divided doses Genotype 2 and 3–800 mg/day in two divided doses
Ribavirin	For sofobuvir based regimes: 1000 mg/day if < 75 kg or 1200 mg/day if ≥ 75 kg in two divided doses
Sofosbuvir	400 mg once a day

Table 8.10: Newer directly acting antiviral

Class of drug	Drugs	Features
Protease inhibitor	Boceprevir Telaprevir Simeprevir	High potency Limited genotypic coverage Low barrier to resistance Drug-drug interaction
NS5A inhibitors	Ledipasvir Daclatasvir	High potency Multi-genotypic coverage Intermediate barrier resistance
NS5B nucleotide (HCV polemerase) inhibitor	Sofosbuvir	High potency Pan-genotypic coverage High barrier to resistance
NS5B non nucleotide inhibitor	Dasabuvir	Intermediate potency Limited genotypic coverage Low barrier to resistance

Summary of AASLD/IDSA Recommendations for HCV Treatment

1. Treatment of therapy-naïve and relapsed patients with genotype 1 HCV infection

Interferon Eligibility	Recommended Regimens	Alternative Regimens
Eligible	Sofosbuvir + peginterferon + ribavirin for 12 wk	Simeprevir for 12 wk + peginterferon + ribavirin for 24 wk
Ineligible	Sofosbuvir + simeprevir ± ribavirin for 12 wk	Sofosbuvir + ribavirin for 24 wk

2. Treatment of patients with genotype 1 HCV infection and non-response to previous therapy

HCV genotype	Recommended regimens	Alternative regimens
Patients in whom prior peginterferon + ribavirin failed		
1	Sofosbuvir + simeprevir ± ribavirin for 12 wk	• Sofosbuvir for 12 wk + peginterferon + ribavirin for 12–24 wk • Simeprevir for 12 wk + peginterferon + ribavirin for 48 wk • Ineligible to receive interferon: Sofosbuvir +ribavirin for 24 wk
Patients in whom prior peginterferon + ribavirin + telaprevir or boceprevir failed		
1	Sofosbuvir for 12 wk + peginterferon + ribavirin for 12–24 wk	• Sofosbuvir + peginterferon + ribavirin for 24 wk • Ineligible to receive interferon: Sofosbuvir +ribavirin for 24 wk

3. Treatment of patients with genotype 2 HCV infection

Population	Recommended regimens	Alternative regimens
Therapy-naive and relapsed patients	Sofosbuvir+ ribavirin for 12 wk	None
Nonresponse to previous therapy	Sofosbuvir + ribavirin for 12 wk	Sofosbuvir + peginterferon +ribavirin for 12 wk

4. Treatment of patients with genotype 3 HCV infection

HCV genotype	Recommended regimens	Alternative regimens
Therapy-naive and relapsed patients	Sofosbuvir + ribavirin for 24 wk	Sofosbuvir + peginterferon +ribavirin for 12 wk
Nonresponse to previous therapy	Sofosbuvir + ribavirin for 24 wk	Sofosbuvir + peginterferon +ribavirin for 12 wk

5. Treatment of treatment naïve or failure of PEG- IFN and ribavirin combination in genotype 4, 5 and 6

HCV genotype	Recommended regimens	Alternative regimens
Genotype 4	Sofosbuvir + ribavirin for 24 wk	Sofosbuvir + peginterferon +ribavirin for 12 wk
Genotype 5 or 6	Sofosbuvir + ledipasvir for 12 wk	Sofosbuvir + peginterferon +ribavirin for 12 wk

Flowchart 8.1: Accidental exposure to blood report to responsible department for assessment of risk immediately after cleaning and rinsing blood on exposed parts. If sample source is negative for both HBAg and anti-HCV then no further action is needed. If source is positive for HBsAg then assess vaccination status of HCW. If unvaccinated or anti-HBS < 10 mIU/ml then take HBIG and HBV vaccine complete course. If source is anti-HCV positive then check anti-HCV after 1 and 3 months. If anti-HCV is still positive then consider treatment for HCV. If anti-HBS >10 mIU/ml or anti-HCV is negative then no further action is required. HBIG: hepatitis B immunoglobulin, HBsAg: hepatitis B surface antigen, HBV: hepatitis B virus, HCV: hepatitis C virus, HCW: health care worker.

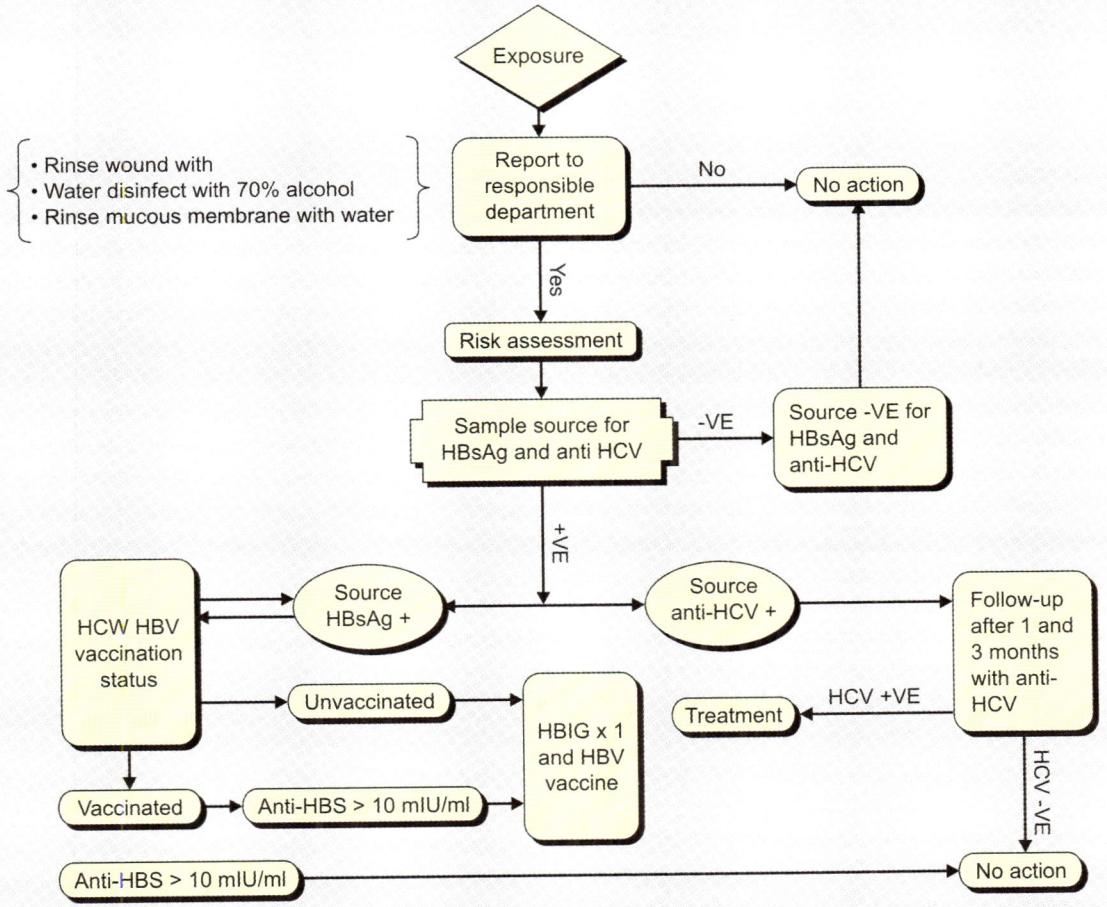

Chronic hepatitis B (CHB) and chronic hepatitis C (CHC) infection remains a serious health care issue in India. Due to awareness programs for HIV and incorporation of Hep B in national immunization schedule, HBsAg prevalence is decreasing particularly among children and adolescents in some part of the country. However, accessibility to treatment remains a significant challenge for many chronically infected patients in India. High cost and lack of reimbursement are the driving factors limiting effective diagnosis and treatment of CHB and CHC in India. There is a need for cost-effective analyses to determine the screening of the risk groups and treatment of these patients.

9

Alcoholic Hepatitis

Shamshersingh Chauhan and Alaka Deshpande

World Health Organization (WHO) estimates that about 2 billion people worldwide consume alcoholic beverages and 76.3 million have diagnosable alcohol-use disorders.

The per capita consumption of alcohol in India has risen to 4 litres per year although it is still less than in US (16.2 litres per year).

50% cases of cirrhosis in India may be due to alcohol abuse.

A high daily intake of alcohol (>60 g in males and >20 g in females) taken for more than 6 to 8 years significantly increases risk of alcoholic liver disease (ALD). Indians develop cirrhosis with smaller quantity and duration of alcohol intake.

A standard drink is equal to 10 grams or 12.5 ml of pure alcohol. Generally, this amount of pure alcohol is found in

- 250 ml of beer
- 100 ml of wine
- 30 ml distilled spirits or liquor (e.g. gin, rum, vodka, or whisky)

Table 9.1: Content and quantity of alcohol in different alcoholic beverages alcohol serving quantity content size of alcohol

	(per cent)	*(in mL)*	*(in grams)*
Beer	5	350	14
Wine	12	120	11
Hard liquor	40	30	10.0

Binge drinking. Binge drinking is defined as a pattern of alcohol consumption that brings the blood alcohol concentration (BAC) level to 0.08% or more. This pattern of drinking usually corresponds to 5 or more drinks on a single occasion for men or 4 or more drinks on a single occasion for women, generally within about 2 hours.

Alcoholic hepatitis is a syndrome of progressive inflammatory liver injury associated with long-term heavy intake of ethanol.

Pathogenesis of Alcohol Induced Liver Injury

The pathogenesis can be explained by three stages in the generation of alcohol induced liver injury:

1. *Steatosis.* Perivenular loading of hepatocytes with fat, which with ongoing drinking then encompasses all the hepatocytes is the initial mechanism in alcohol induced liver injury. This occurs due to alcohol dehydrogenase and acetaldehyde dehydrogenase, the two enzymes related in the metabolism of alcohol leads to reduction of nicotinamide adenine dinucleotide (NAD) to NADH. The altered ratio of NAD/NADH promotes fatty acid accumulation through the inhibition of gluconeogenesis and fatty acid oxidation. Cessation of drinking at this juncture can reverse this steatosis in almost all people by three weeks. If, however the

drinking continues then the steatosis takes form of steatohepatitis and hepatocyte injury begins.

2. *Inflammation.* Chronic alcoholism can up-regulate the cytochrome P450 enzymes and can affect the metabolism of many drugs. One of these is the cytochrome CYP2E1 which also metabolizes alcohol, like alcohol dehydrogenase and causes formation of acetaldehyde. Increased quantities of acetaldehyde due to chronic alcoholism can lead to formation of protein adducts with the intracellular proteins and interfere in the cellular function. Acetaldehyde-modified proteins and lipids on the cell surface may behave as neo-antigens and trigger immunologic injury. Many free radicals are generated as by-products of ethanol metabolism which add to the cellular injury. In addition, acetaldehyde reacts with glutathione and depletes this key element of the hepatocytic defence against free radicals. Other anti-oxidant defenses, including selenium, zinc, and vitamin E, are often reduced in individuals with alcoholism. Peroxidation of membrane lipids accompanies alcoholic liver injury and may be involved in cell death and inflammation.

The intestinal permeability to endotoxin, produced by colonic flora, is increased in chronic alcoholics. These endotoxins when reach the damaged liver they cannot be effectively cleared. Being pro-inflammatory they induce hepatocyte damage.

3. *Fibrogenesis.* Acetaldehyde protein adducts along with ethanol itself, induce Kuppfer cell activation. Fibrogenic cytokines are produced by them which initiate the unyielding repair process that will ultimately culminate in cirrhosis over years of insult to the liver cells.

Genetic polymorphism of the cytochrome enzymes (that is why some people are more susceptible to alcohol induced liver injury than others), deficiency of antioxidants in an already malnourished chronic alcoholic, concomitant hepatitis B and hepatitis C infection in these high-risk behaviour individuals also increase the hepatocyte damage.

Although 90% to 100% of heavy drinkers show evidence of fatty livers, only 10% to 35% develop alcoholic hepatitis and 5% to 15% develop cirrhosis.

Clinical Features

Alcoholic hepatitis has a large spectrum. At one end is totally asymptomatic patient with mild aminotransferase elevation detected on routine check-up to a patient with hepatic encephalopathy, coagulopathy and portal hypertension without liver cirrhosis.

A typical history depicting alcohol abuse with symptoms related to chronic liver disease can be attributed to alcohol induced liver injury.

Alcohol abuse can be identified using a structured questionnaire such as the alcohol use disorders identification test (AUDIT) or more easily the CAGE (Cut-down, annoyed, feeling guilty and alcohol as an eye opener) questionnaire or the rapid alcohol problems screen (RAPS) questionnaire.

Patients with clinically symptomatic alcoholic hepatitis typically present with non-specific symptoms of nausea, malaise, and low-grade fever. Anaemia may be present due to malnutrition, GI losses, etc. The liver is usually enlarged, often with mild tenderness. Hepatomegaly results from both steatosis and swelling of injured hepatocytes. Mild right upper quadrant discomfort can be present. A bruit can be heard over the liver in more than 50% of the cases in severe alcoholic hepatitis.

Manifestations of hepatic failure or portal hypertension may include scleral icterus with darkening of the urine, splenomegaly, asterixis (a flapping tremor characteristic of metabolic encephalopathies), peripheral oedema, and bulging flanks with shifting abdominal dullness (indicating the presence of ascites).

Spider angiomata, proximal muscle wasting, altered hair distribution, and gynaecomastia may be observed, although these findings most commonly reflect co-existent cirrhosis.

Factors associated with increased mortality:
a. Older age
b. Acute kidney injury concomitantly associated
c. High discriminant score
d. Leucocytosis
e. Alcohol consumption >120 g/day
f. Presence of sepsis
g. Ratio of total bilirubin to gamma glutamyl-transferase >1
h. Neutrophil to lymphocyte ratio >4.

Investigations

The ALT is typically less than the AST in alcohol induced liver injury. This is because alcohol induces deficiency of pyridoxal phosphate required for ALT formation. AST is usually below 400 IU/L and ALT is usually below 100–120 IU/L. Gammaglutamyl transferase is also elevated but not specific for alcohol induced liver injury. Alkaline phosphatase may be normal or slightly elevated (<3 times upper normal limit). Serum bilirubin may be markedly raised. Hypoalbuminemia reveals a chronic and serious disease.

Severe alcoholic hepatitis can be diagnosed when prothrombin time is delayed >5 sec, anaemia, hypoalbuminaemia, serum bilirubin more than 8 mg/dl, leucocytosis with increased polymorphonuclear cells >5500/cumm and presence of encephalopathy, renal failure and ascites.

Ultrasonography can quantify the hepatomegaly with Doppler studies showing increased peak systolic pressure in hepatic artery.

The Maddrey's discriminant function calculated as 4.6 × (Pt's prothrombin time in secs-control prothrombin time in secs) + serum total bilirubin can be used to prognosticate the patients. A score of >32 depicts poor prognosis. A score more than 54 may classify the patient as non-responder to treatment. Also the model for end stage liver disease, the MELD score using INR, serum total bilirubin and serum creatinine with a score more than 21 shows poor prognosis.

A new score, Glasgow alcoholic hepatitis score is formed which takes into account the

Age <50 years (1 point); >50 years (2 points)

Total WBCs <15000/mm^3 (1point) >15000/mm^3 (2 points)

Blood urea <14 mg/dl (1point); >14 mg/dl (2 points)

INR < 1.5 (1 point) 1.5–2 (2 points) > 2 (3 points)

Total bilirubin:
<7.3 mg/dl (1 point) 7.3–14.6 mg/dl (2 points) > 14.6 mg/dl (3 points)

Patients having a score more than 9 show benefit with treatment of the condition with corticosteroids.

The likely hood of underlying cirrhosis can be assessed by elastography which can show the evidence of increased liver stiffness due to oedema and fibrosis.

Biopsy of the liver is usually not indicated in every case for diagnosis but in doubtful cases it can be done, especially through the transvenous route (due to presence of coagulopathies). It shows micro and macro-vesicularsteatosis (similar to nonalcoholic steatohepatitis (NASH) with predominant neutrophillic infiltration in the surrounding parenchyma. Mallory Denk bodies (MDB) may be seen in the damaged hepatocytes (other conditions where these bodies are seen are Indian childhood cirrhosis, starvation, NASH, post-jejunal bypass, use of amiodarone).

Differential Diagnosis

Acute viral hepatitis, acute Budd-Chiari syndrome, drug induced especially paracetamol which in therapeutic doses in chronic alcoholics can cause liver damage, non-alcoholic steato-hepatitis, ischaemic hepatitis, autoimmune hepatitis, Wilson's disease.

Treatment

In most patients with alcoholic hepatitis, the illness is mild. Their short-term prognosis is good, and no specific treatment is required. Providing supplemental vitamins and minerals, including folate and thiamine, is reasonable. The treatment depends on the stage of the disease and presence of complications of hepatic cirrhosis, such as GI bleed, ascites or encephalopathy. It includes certain general measures and specific treatment.

General Measures

Abstinence

This is the cornerstone of management. Abstinence improves survival, improves hepatic histology, reduces portal pressure and progression to cirrhosis. Baclofen may aid in abstinence.

Nutritional Support

There is a high prevalence of protein-calorie malnutrition in patients with ALD. The degree of malnutrition correlates directly with mortality.

In general, enteral nutrition is preferable over parenteral supplementation. Protein should be supplied (1 to 1.5 g/kg body weight/day) to provide positive nitrogen balance. Patients may also have depletion of potassium, magnesium and phosphates which may require replacement. Patients who are coagulopathic should receive vitamin K parenterally. Alcohol withdrawal symptoms may be anticipated and managed appropriately. Gastric acid suppression with proton pump inhibitors, sucralfate is helpful.

Specific Drug Therapy

Patients with severe acute alcoholic hepatitis are at high-risk of early death, at a rate of 50% or greater within 30 days, the strongest factor predictive of short-term mortality is hepatic encephalopathy.

In patients with severe disease (Maddrey discriminant function [MDF] score >32),

unless steroids are contraindicated, prednisolone should be considered. Prednisolone at 40 mg per day for 4 weeks and then tapered over four weeks is the standard therapy. Patients with mild forms of alcoholic hepatitis should not be treated with steroids.

A Lilles's score is calculated at the end of day 7 of steroid treatment to look for response to steroid treatment. A score ≥0.45 predicts poor prognosis and requires different forms of treatment.

Alternative approved treatment to severe alcoholic hepatitis is pentoxfylline 400 mg three times daily for 4 weeks. Pentoxifylline may be considered, especially if prednisolone cannot be used in presence of pancreatitis, GI bleeding, renal failure, sepsis, etc.

It has significant anti-TNF activity and hence suppresses inflammation. It is also shown to decrease the risk of hepatorenal syndrome.

Lenalidomide at a dose of 10 mg daily has shown to be effective in many trials for severe alcoholic hepatitis. It is a very potent tumour necrosis factor (TNF) alpha antagonist, more potent than pentoxiphylline for alcoholic hepatitis. If Maddreys score is more than 54 then lenadilomide is the drug to be used. Thromboembolism, bone marrow suppression, hepatotoxicity limit its use in certain settings.

Other drugs like N-acetyl cysteine, anabolic steroids, colchicine have limited use. Infliximab and etenacept have been associated with deaths and are not used.

Lactulose, rifaximin and norfloxacin may be used as gut decontaminants to decrease endotoxin production.

Liver Transplantation in Alcoholic Liver Disease

Acute alcoholic hepatitis, no matter how severe, is a contraindication for liver transplantation. Patients with end-stage ALD should be considered for liver transplant. Generally, 6 months of abstinence is considered necessary as eligibility for liver transplantation.

10

Autoimmune Hepatitis

Alaka Deshpande

Autoimmune hepatitis (AIH) is an inflammatory liver disease associated with positive auto-antibodies, hypergammaglobulinaemia, plasma cell infiltrate of the liver. It is a diagnosis by exclusion as the term is poorly defined. In 1940s,Waldenstrom recognized the relevance of hypergammaglobulinaemia in chronic hepatitis. Autoimmune hepatitis is appreciated since then in young females with persistent liver disease as well as extra-hepatic manifestations like rash, arthralgia, ammenorrhoea and fever. The serological diagnosis in those days was not feasible. But today laboratory findings suggestive of autoimmunity and response to the immune suppressive therapy like steroids and azathioprine prompted Cowling and Mackay in 1965 to use this term and in 1993 the auto-immune hepatitis has been endorsed globally.

Pathogenesis of Autoimmune Hepatitis

Like other autoimmune disorders, the environmental agent triggers the autoimmune process in a genetically predisposed individual resulting in loss of tolerance to self-antigens. The precise genetic predisposition and its relationship remain speculative.

The environmental triggers vary widely including infectious agents *viz.* hepatitis viruses, other viruses having long latency, immuniza-tions, herbs, drugs, etc. but in most cases the specific trigger/inducer of auto-immunity cannot be identified at a time when patient presents with AIH.

Mechanisms may be:

1. Molecular mimicry
2. Exposure of sequestered antigen
3. Altered self-antigen
4. Neo-antigen formed by a combination of foreign determinant and self-antigen.

Clinical Features

Female preponderance is seen. However, the disease is seen in both sexes and all age groups. The clinical spectrum varies from asymptomatic to cirrhosis.Patient is asymptomatic but persistence of raised aminotransferases may initiate other labo-ratory investigations. About one-third of patients present with acute hepatitis which is indistinguishable from viral hepatitis. Half of the patients may have chronic hepatitis.

Symptomatic patients frequently complain of fatigue, arthritis, arthralgia, acne, and ammenorrhoea. Patients may present with acute liver failure. Many patients diagnosed as cryptogenic cirrhosis at presentation may include cases without detectable auto-antibodies. Majority of the patients may have antecedent subclinical disease.

Other autoimmune diseases particularly Sjögren's syndrome, auto-immune thyroid

Variable	Cut-off	Points	Cut-off	Points
Table 10.1: Shows simplified diagnostic criteria for autoimmune hepatitis (AIH)				
ANA or SMA	≥ 1:40	1	≥ 1:80	2
or LKM	—	—	≥ 1:40	2
or SLA positive	—	—	—	2
IgG	> ULN	1	> 1.1 ULN	2
Histology	Compatible	1	Typical	2
Absenceof viral hepatitis	—	—	Yes	2

Six (6) points probable → AIH
More than seven (7) points → Definitive AIH

disease, autoimmune haemolysis, rheumatoid arthritis, ulcerative colitis, ITP, may be associated with AIH.

Laboratory Features

Elevated levels of aspartate aminotransferase, and alkaline phosphatase are noted. Hyper-bilirubinaemia, hypoalbuminaemia, and coagulopathy are seen in acute presentations.

Serological Markers

Anti-nuclear antibody (ANA) alone is detected in 10% of cases. Half of the patients have ANA with smooth muscle antibody (SMA) present. ANA and SMA levels fluctuate during the course of AIH and may disappear with corticosteroid therapy.

Patients with antiliver-kidney microsome-1 (ALKM-1), antiliver cytosol-1 (ALC-1) along with AIH are classified as AIH type 2.

Liver biopsy. Histologic appearance is that of chronic hepatitis with mononuclear cell infiltrate. Abundance of plasma cells, eosino-phils which invade the sharply demarcated hepatocyte boundary (limiting plate), piece meal necrosis, bridging necrosis are evident on histopathology.

Variant Syndromes

Autoimmune hepatitis—primary biliary cirrhosis: AIH-PBC have characteristic clinical, logical and histological findings of both the diseases.

AIH-PSC: (Primary Sclerosing cholangitis) have serologic and histologic features of AIH and cholangiographic characteristics of PSC.

Management: AIH in general is steroid responsive. It is not possible to suggest standard treatment protocol in view of paucity of clinical trials.

The initial regimen may be prednisolone 60 mg/day tapered off over a month to a maintenance dose of 20 mg/day or Predni-solone 30 mg/day + Azathioprine 50 mg/day has also been effective. Prednisolone is tapered off to 10 mg/day over a month while azathioprine is continued in the same dose. In cases refractory to these regimens other immunosuppresants are tried. If patient progresses to cirrhosis or its complications then liver transplant is the only recourse.

Presentation after Liver Transplant

AIH can occur *de novo* after liver transplant (so called alloimmune hepatitis) or recur in those transplanted for AIH.

11

Drug
Induced Hepatitis

Alaka Deshpande

Better understanding of the disease processes has facilitated development of newer drugs as the therapeutic targets are being defined. However, large number of molecules in pipeline of drug development are rejected because of drug induced liver injury (DILI).

Genetic predisposition, other biological factors, ethnic diversity, pre-existing insults of the liver and idiosyncracies contribute to DILI.

The liver injury may follow drug inhalation, ingestion, parenteral administration, and topical application.

The drugs include prescribed therapeutic agents, drugs available over the counter (OTC), herbal, other alternate medicines, a large number of organic and inorganic compounds which may be ingested accidentally or intentionally.

Liver injury is caused by medicinal drugs, nutritional products or molecules used for recreational purposes. Combination of drugs or simultaneous use of multiple drugs can enhance hepatotoxicity, e.g. rifampicin induced INH toxicity. The pre-existing affectation of the liver by alcohol, viral agents like HBV, HCV, IV drug abuse further add to the insult.

Two major types of hepatotoxicity are recognized 1. Direct toxicity, 2. Idiosyncratic.

The liver plays a major role in drug metabolism (Fig 11.1). It depends on the the

pharmacokinetics of the drug *viz.* efficiency of the drug metabolizing enzymes, intrinsic clearance, binding to plasma proteins and the hepatic blood flow.

The metabolism can produce an active metabolite or degradation product. The drugs are eliminated by kidney if the end product is water soluble. But if the drug is lipid soluble then it is converted from lipid soluble to water soluble substance that can be excreted into urine or bile.

Mechanism of Liver Injury

1. Inhibition of mitochondrial function which prevents fatty acid metabolism and results into accumulation of reactive oxygen species and lactates.
2. Disruption of intracellular calcium homeostasis.
3. Induction of apoptosis.
4. Drug-enzyme complex forms a nonfunctional adducts which leads to presentation on the cell surface of hepatocytes as new immunogens which are attacked by T-lymphocytes.
5. Disruption of bile canalicular transport mechanisms.

The microsomal fraction of hepatocyte's endoplasmic reticulum has the drug metabolizing system. The oxidation and hydroxylation processes with the help of enzyme system degrade the drug. They have mixed functions.

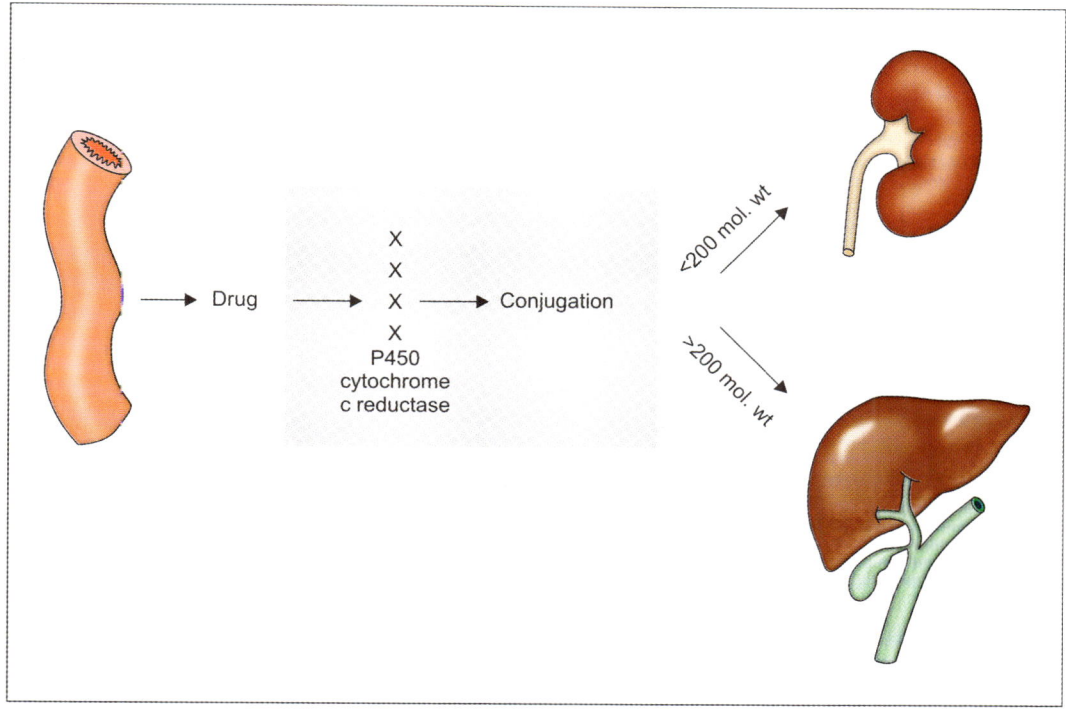

Fig. 11.1: Drug metabolism

The monoxygenases, cytochrome C reductase and cytochrome P450 system play the major role. In addition, alcoholic dehydrogenase, glucuronidase, sulfotransferase, etc. conjugate the drugs enhancing their solubility.

Active transport of drugs takes place at the biliary pole of the hepatocytes. Many factors decide whether the drugs will be eliminated via urine or bile or both.

Forms of Drug Induced Liver Injuries

- Acute hepatitis
- Steatohepatitis
- Cholestasis
- Granulomatous hepatitis
- Drug induced chronic hepatitis
- Hepatic fibrosis
- Hepatic adenomas

Score	Grade	Definition
		Table 11.1: Severity of drug induced hepatitis
1.	Mild	↑ ALT, S, Bil <2.5 mg/dl INR <1.5
2.	Moderate	↑ ALT, *S. Bilirubin* >2.5 mg/dl, INR >1.5
3.	Moderate-severe	ALT, bilirubin, INR Increased + patient hospitalized because of liver injury induced by drug
4.	Severe	All the above + one of the following 1 Hepatic failure (ascites, encephalopathy) 1 Other organ failure due to liver injury
5.	Fatal	Liver transplantation because of liver injury or death.

Table 11.2: Shows commonly used drugs and chemicals and their hepatotoxicity

A drug may have more than one type of liver injuries

Hepatitis	Halothane, isonex, rifampicin, pyrazinamide, nitrofurantoin, phenobarbitone, carbamazpine, valproic acid, methyldopa, enalapril, lisinopril, losartan, nifedipine, verapamil, diltiazem, Ibuprofen, indomethacin, diclofenac, antifungal drugs, AZT, stavudine, nevirapine, indinavir, tipranavir.
Cholestasis	Methyltestosterone, carbamazepine, clopidogrel, cyclosporine Ezetimibe, methimazole, chlorpromazine, tricyclic antidepressants.
Fatty liver	Amiodarone, valproic acid, methotrexate, asparaginase, indinavir, tetracycline
Granulomas	Sulphonamides, carbamazepine, quinidine, allopurinol.
Liver necrosis	Acetaminophen, carbon tetrachloride, yellow phosphorus

Table 11.3

Herbal remedy	Indication	Pattern of liver injury
Atractylis gummifera	Purgative, emetic	Acute liver failure
Camphor	Rubefacient	Abnormal liver test, encephalopathy
Carp capsules	Rheumatism	Abnormal liver enzymes, liver necrosis in rats
Cascara sagrada	Laxative	Cholestasis
Chaparral leaf	Multiple uses	Massive necrosis, chronic hepatitis
Chaso	Slimming aid	Massive necrosis, hepatitis
Lipokinetix	Slimming aid	Acute hepatitis, acute liver failure
Usnic acid	Slimming aid	Acute liver failure
Dai-saiko-to	Chronic hepatitis	Acute and chronic hepatitis
Greater celandine	Gallstone	Acute hepatitis, fibrosis, cholestasis
"Green juice"	Dietary suppliment	Granulomatous hepatitis
Green tea extracts (exolise, etc.)		
Herbal tea	Accute hepatocellular injury	
Herbal life	Health suppliment	Acute hepatitis cholestasis
Isabgol	Laxative	Giant cell hepatitis (one report)
Kava	Anxiety disorder	Diffuse hepatocellular necrosis
Lycopodium similiaplex	Insomnia	Acute hepatitis
Margosa oil	Health tonic	Reye's syndrome
Oil of cloves	Dental pain	Zonal necrosis (dose dependent)

The drug induced liver injury network (DILIN) has developed a grading system for severity of liver disease.

Management

The detailed history of exposure to chemicals or drugs of all types in preceding three months is essential so that in case of drug induced liver injury, the offending agent has to be discontinued **immediately**.

Supportive care is given, majority of the cases recover depending on the severity of the toxicity.

12

HIV Disease and the Liver

Alaka Deshpande

The devastating effects of HIV pandemic are seen over last three decades. HIV infection per se or the opportunistic infections due to immune deficiency and the drug therapy affect all the various organs in the body. Liver is no exception.

The involvement of liver in AIDS is usually an indicator of disseminated disease. A host of aetiological agents such as mycobacteria, candida, cryptococci, microsporidia, toxoplasma, leishmania, peliosis, cytomegalovirus (CMV) as well as non-diagnostic markers of liver involvement such as macrosteatosis, granulomas, etc. have been widely reported in liver biopsy studies.

In developing countries including India the most common route of HIV acquisition is unprotected multipartner heterosexual activity, followed by IV drug use (IVDU), men having sex with men (MSM) and vertical transmission.

In addition to these risk factors, large number of these cases are chronic alcoholics which itself results into liver injury.

HBV and HCV infections are also acquired by the same risk behaviour. Large number of co-infected cases of HIV-HBV and HIV-HCV remain undetected because of ignorance, marginalization of this community reluctant to come forward for testing and paucity of testing facilities.

The liver involvement of liver in HIV disease is mainly due to:
1. Chronic HIV infection, associated malnutrition, alcoholism
2. Opportunistic infections due to immune deficiency
3. Co-infections like HBV, HCV
4. HIV related malignancies
5. Drug therapy.

Steatosis. Steatosis is an abnormal accumulation of triglycerides and other lipids in hepatocytes. It is due to multifactorial defects in lipid metabolism. Figs 12.1 and 12.2 show steatosis.

Chronic HIV infection, malnutrition, lack of hepatoprotective dietary substances *per se* can be responsible for these changes. ARV

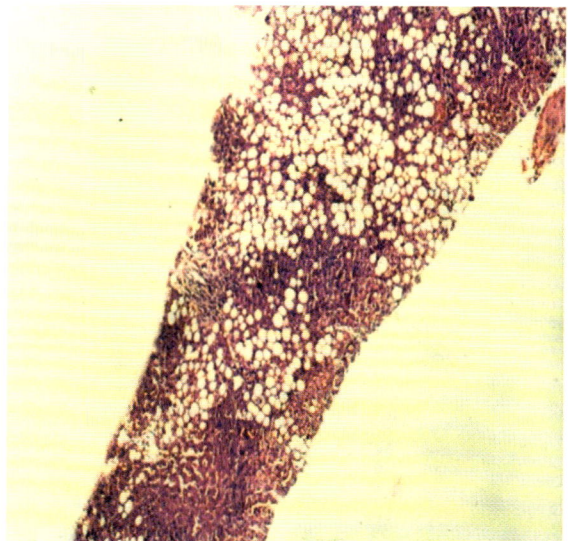

Fig. 12.1: Macrosteatosis-low power, H and E stain

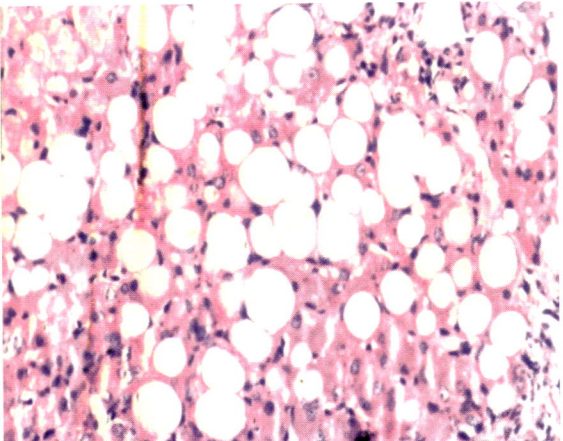

Fig. 12.2: Macrosteatosis under HP

drugs particularly stavudine have also been incriminated for these changes.

Opportunistic Infections (OI)

Bacterial infections. Tuberculosis is the most common opportunistic infections (OI) in HIV disease in India. The liver is affected by TB as a part of disseminated TB, TB lymphnodes in porta hepatis or hepatic tuberculomas.

The patient may present with unexplained fever, hepatomegaly, raised alkaline phosphatase. The liver biopsy reveals granulomas with AFBs. In advanced immune deficiency state (CD$_4$<50) mycobacterium avium complex affects various organs (Figs 12.3 and 12.4).

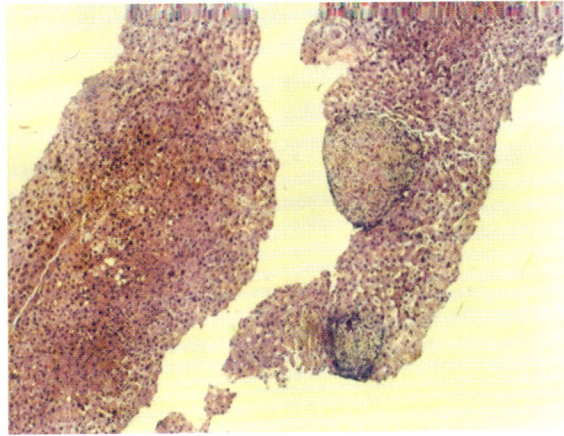

Fig. 12.3: Two kissing granulomas seen under LP–H and E

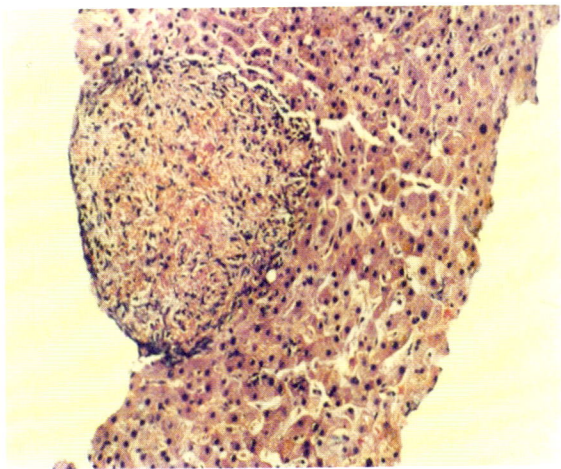

Fig. 12.4: Large granuloma without caseation HP, H and E

Peliosis

Peliosis hepatis. It is an uncommon vascular condition characterised by randomly distributed multiple blood-filled cavities throughout the liver. The size of the cavities usually varies between a few millimeters to 3 cm in diameter.

Microscopically, two different types of peliosis can be distinguished in the liver: (1) "parenchymal peliosis" consisting of irregular cavities that are neither lined by sinusoidal cells nor by fibrous tissue, and (2) "phlebectatic peliosis" characterized by regular, spherical cavities lined by endothelium and/or fibrosis.

Prior to AIDS, peliosis hepatis had been rarely reported as a consequence of chronic infections such as tuberculosis, advanced malignancy or steroid/azathioprine therapy. Ultrastructural studies done previously comparing HIV associated peliosis with non-HIV peliosis using Warthin-Starry stain, noted a gram-negative bacillus in the cystic spaces. DNA studies designated this bacillus as *Rochalimaea henselae* which induces peliotic changes. Scoazec described a peculiar feature of the presence of hyperplastic sinusoidal macrophages suggesting that endothelial cell injury may precipitate these sinusoidal changes (Figs 12.5 and 12.6).

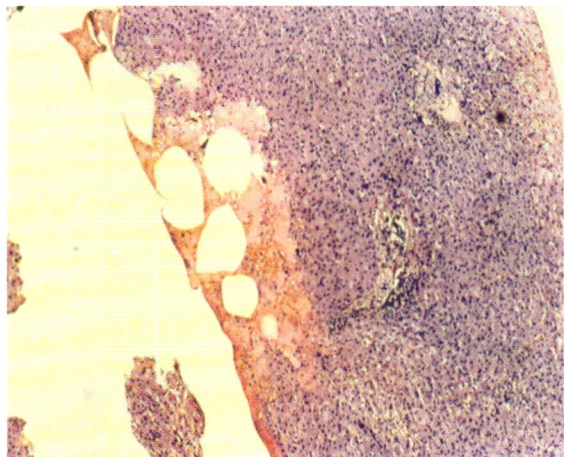

Fig. 12.5: Peliosis hepatis

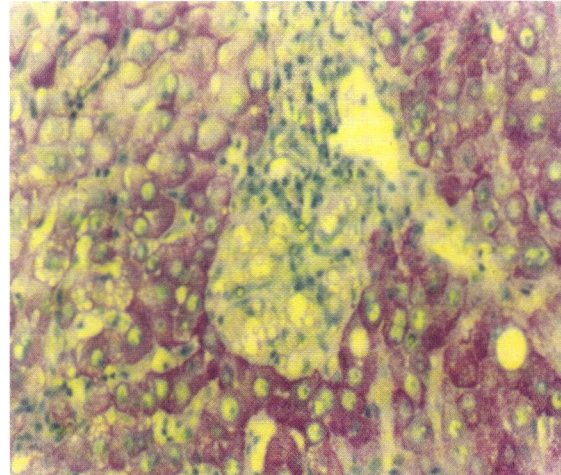

Fig. 12.7: Cryptococci seen under LP-PAS

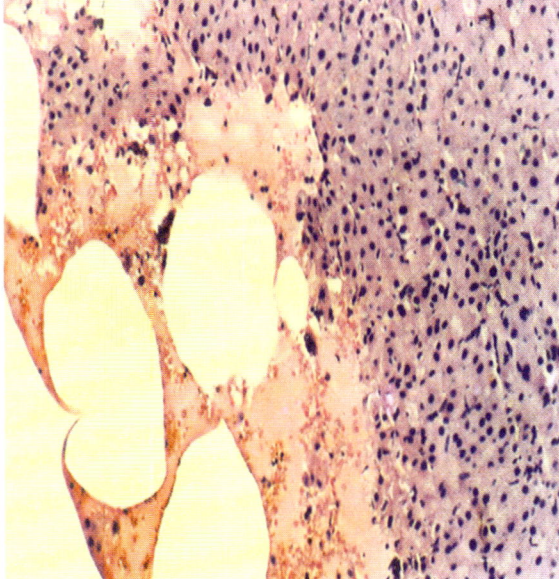

Fig. 12.6: Blood filled spaces not lined by endothelial cells

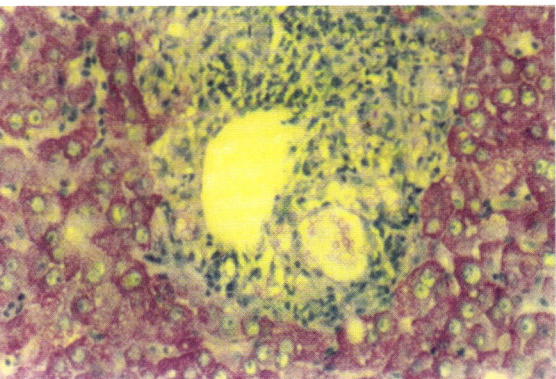

Fig. 12.8: Cryptococci-spherical bodies seen under HP-PAS

Fungal infections. Histoplasmosis, *cryptococcus neoformans*, *Coccidiodomycosis*, *Candida albicans* are fungii which affect the liver in severe immunodeficiency. The patient may present with unexplained low grade fever, hepatomegaly and raised transaminases. Liver may be involved as a part of the systemic fungal infection.

Figures 12.7 and 12.8 show hepatic cryptococcoma. The microscopy confirmed the fungal infection. Liver involvement by *Cryptococcus neoformans* indicates disseminated infection of *C. neoformans*.

Parasitic infections. Multiple amoebic abscesses are commonly seen in our country. Toxoplasmosis also presents as multiple focal lesions.

Hepatitis. Hepatitis due to other viral infections, alcoholism, and drug induced hepatitis is common in presence of HIV disease. Infiltration with inflammatory cells is evident Fig. 12.9).

Viral infections. Apart from HIV-HBV and HIV-HCV co-infections, other viruses like CMV, varicella zoster, Epstein-Barr virus cause liver injury.

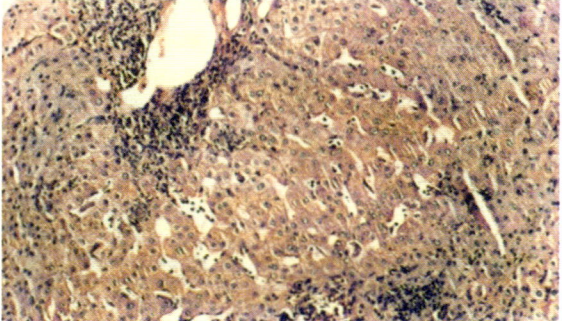

Fig. 12.9: Acute hepatitis, inflammatory cell infiltrate, H and E stain

CO-INFECTIONS: HIV-HBV, HIV-HCV

HIV and HBV share common risk factors for transmission. Worldwide more than 4 million individuals are estimated to be co-infected. Prior exposure to HBV can be found in about 90 % of HIV cases. The prevalence of chronic HBV infection in HIV is around 10 %. Various studies have shown 3 to 14 times higher morbidity and mortality in HIV- HBV infected cases.

It is recommended that testing for HBV infection should be the part of initial evaluation of all HIV infected cases. A patient positive for HbsAg, HBV DNA, HbeAg and anti-HbeAg characterizes the status of the infection.

Co-infected cases have higher HBV viral load and lower levels of serum ALT compared to only HBV infected cases.

HIV accelerates progression to cirrhosis, ESLD and HCC.

WHO guidelines recommend cARV (combination of anti-retroviral) therapy for co-infected cases irrespective of CD4 counts.

HBV being an immune-mediated infection, immune damage of the liver may occur after immune reconstitution following HAART.

Tenofovir (TDF) and lamivudine (LMV) are potent agents against both the viruses. Regular monitoring of both viral loads is necessary once the therapy is initiated.

Longevity of HIV cases has increased in post HAART era so also the morbidity related to liver diseases and hepatocellular carcinoma (HCC).

HBV vaccine. HIV-infected individual having all the HBV markers negative should receive HBV vaccine. The anti-HBV antibody response will depend on the severity of immunodeficiency so after vaccination anti-HBs antibody evaluation is necessary as the antibody response in immunodeficiency is unpredictable.

HIV-HCV coinfection. An estimated 170 million people are HCV infected worldwide and about 4 to 5 million people are co-infected with HIV.

Both the viruses are single stranded RNA viruses with a very high rate of replication and both the viruses evade the host-immune system due to a high genetic variability 0.25 to 30 % of HIV infected cases are coinfected with HCV. Although HCV infection is not efficiently transmitted in heterosexual relationship, recent reports show transmission in MSMs. HCV testing should be the part of initial evaluation of HIV case.

The coinfection increases the liver related morbidity. The prolonged longevity in post HAART era has resulted into rising incidence of HCC. The drug interaction between the ART and anti HCV therapy need to be seriously considered before initiation of therapy.

Liver transplant in these co-infected cases is a promising option however proper selection of the case ensures the success. One has to consider controlled HIV viral load, CD4 > 200, interactios between ARVs and post-transplant immunosuppressants. It requires a multidisciplinary approach.

HIV associated neoplasms. Primary as well as metastatic non-Hodgkin's lymphoma is common malignant neoplasm associated with HIV. Kaposi's sarcoma is rare in India. With increased longevity after anti-retroviral therapy, patients with HCV, HBV co-infections may develop hepatocellular carcinoma.

Antiretroviral Therapy and Liver

Drug induced liver injury (DILI) is increasingly impacting the clinical practice. The drugs may be directly hepatotoxic or may be inducers of hepatic cytochrome P450 enzyme system.

HIV patient in addition to anti-retreoviral therapy may be receiving large number of drugs either as a prophylaxis or treatment of OI. The protease inhibitor indinavir (IDV), fortovase (FTV), etc. are metabolized by liver with enzyme induction, the drug level either of ARVs or other drugs may be affected. For example, serum concentration of protease inhibitors and drug interaction.

	Indinavir (IDV) ARV-protease inhibitor	Fortovase (FTV) ARV-protease inhibitor
Ketoconazole	↑ 68%	↑ X3
Rifampicin	↓ 89%	↓ 34%
Rifabutin	↓ 32%	↓ 40%
Oral contraceptives	OC ↑	Nodata
Lipid lowering agents	LL ↑	LL ↑

Ketoconazole increases serum concentration of IDV and FTV thereby may increase the toxicity of these drugs. As against, anti TB drugs rifampicin and rifabutin lower the serum levels of IDV and FTV thereby may lead to HIV drug resistance.

The concentration of oral contraceptives and lipid lowering agents is increased by these protease inhibitors thereby leading to the toxicity of OCs and lipid lowering agents.

The earlier therapy guidelines included nevirapine in a first-line triple combination ARV therapy. Being hepatotoxic about less than 5% of cases developed jaundice. The revised WHO guidelines of ART therapy has replaced nevirapine by efavirenz.

Indirect hyperbilirubinaemia is a known side-effect of atazanavir therapy which is self-resolving.

13

Nonalcoholic Fatty Liver Disease

Alaka Deshpande

Non-alcoholic fatty liver disease (NAFLD) is one of the most common liver disease world over today. It is becoming the most common cause of chronic liver disease in adults paralleling the epidemic of obesity in developed countries.

It is increasingly being recognized as a hepatic manifestation of insulin resistance and the systemic complex of metabolic syndrome. It is emerging to be the cause of many cases so far known as cryptogenic cirrhosis. It gradually progresses to cirrhosis and even in the absence of cirrhosis may be the cause of hepatocellular carcinoma. It is now one of the leading causes for liver transplant.

Virchow in nineteenth century gave the first scientific account of fatty infiltration of the liver. Morgan in 1870, described an association between obesity and fatty liver. Zelman reported fibrosis and cirrhosis in obese individuals without significant alcohol intake.

Ludwig in 1980 presented his clinical experience in non-alcoholic steatohepatitis (NASH) and named this condition. Since then the renewed interest in this entity has now shown that NASH is the most common cause of cryptogenic cirrhosis which accounts for 10–20% of all cirrhosis.

Definition

It is defined as liver fat content more than 5–10% by weight and frequently more than 5–10% of macrosteatotic hepatocytes.

Terminology

Following is the working classification of NAFLD.

NNFL: Non-NASH fatty liver

Type I NAFLD: Steatosis without inflammation or fibrosis

Type II NAFLD: Steatosis with non-specific lobular inflammation without fibrosis

Or hepatocyte ballooning.

NASH:

Type III NAFLD: Steatosis with inflammation and fibrosis.

Type IV NAFLD: Steatosis, inflammation, hepatocyte ballooning and fibrosis.

CONDITIONS ASSOCIATED WITH NAFLD

- Central/truncal obesity
- Type 2 diabetes mellitus
- Hyperinsulinemia—metabolic syndrome
- Hyperlipidemia
- Hypertension
- Polycystic ovarian syndrome (PCOS)

Polycystic Ovarian Syndrome (PCOS)

- Genetic/metabolic conditions
  - Lipodystrophies
  - Mitochondrial diseases
  - Weber-Christian disease
  - Wilson disease

- Drug Related
  - Methotrexate
  - Tamoxifene
  - Amiodarone
  - Nucleoside analogs—Stavudine, zidovudine
  - Protease inhibitors
  - Solvents and industrial toxins
  - Carbon tetrachloride
  - Ethyl bromide
  - Vinyl chloride
  - Perchlorethylene
  - Petrochemicals
- Nutrition
  - Total parenteral nutrition
  - Severe protein malnutrition
  - Celiac disease

Obesity: Studies report 4 to 6 fold increased risk of fatty liver in obese patients compared to nonobese cases. Study of more than 1600 patients undergoing bariatric surgery, the liver histology revealed NNFL in 85–90%, NASH in 25–30% and unsuspected cirrhosis in 1–2% of cases. Insulin resistance too, is very common in NAFLD.

The factors which influence NAFLD are ethnicity, genetic variation and family history (Fig. 13.1).

NAFLD can be viewed as a condition within the spectrum of the metabolic syndrome and systemic lipotoxicity.

A cascade of events lead to cellular ballooning, cell death, organ fibrosis and cirrhosis. Oxidative injury plays the major role. Oxidative injury involves endoplasmic reticulum and small fat droplets. FFA induces changes in the mitochondrial permeability and activation of apoptosis pathways (caspases), caspase induced cytoskeletal injury (Mallory Denk bodies) and cell death by necrosis and apoptosis. This process activates the stellate cells which produce collagen leading to fibrosis and cirrhosis.

In metabolic syndrome attention is paid to organokines. Liver derived proteins—hepatokines are altered in NAFLD. Various studies have shown that altered hepatokine production is associated with development and progression of NAFLD.

Steatosis: Macrovesicular and microvesicular fat droplets with ballooned hepatocytes

Flowchart 13.1

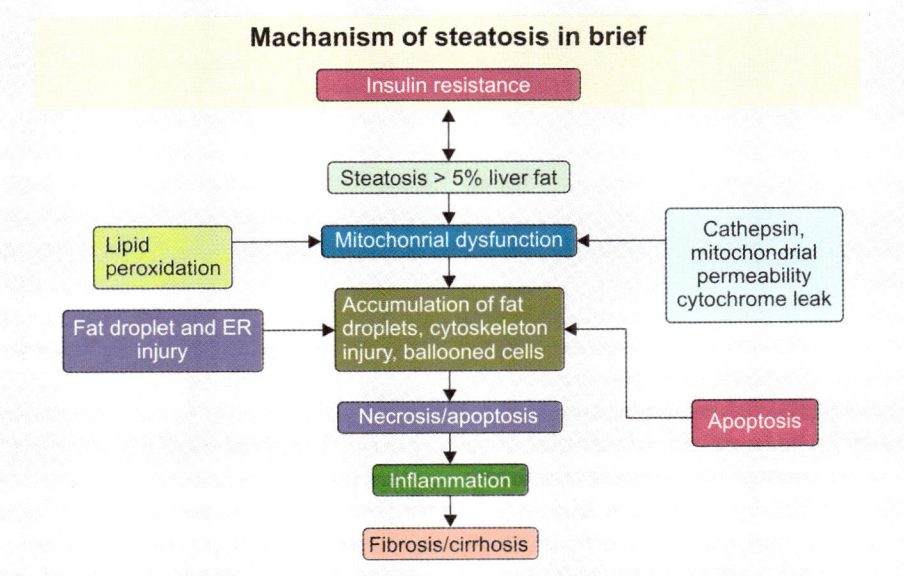

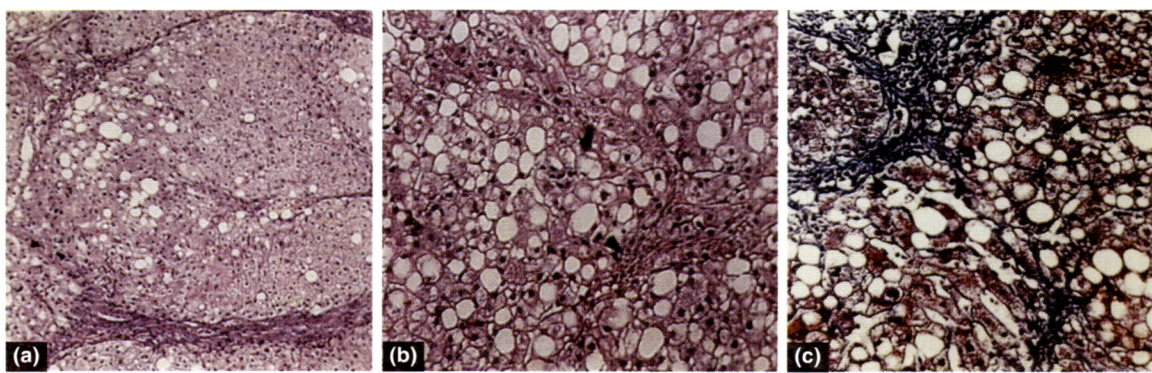

Fig. 13.1: A 65 yrs old female patient obese, diabetic liver biopsy showing steatohepatitis with cirrhosis. Pictures B and C are biopsy specimen of the son of the first patient with mild obesity without diabetes with raised liver enzymes showing NASH (B-H & E stain). These slides also illustrate a familial pattern seen in about 20% of cases.

containing dense, central nuclei sparing the periportal zone is seen. Hepatocytes have a foamy appearance, often containing Mallory-Denk bodies and fibrosis. Although all the scoring systems of NASH have included ballooning of hepatocytes as an important histological parameter, the consensus definition has remained elusive.

Insulin resistance is seen in majority of cases of NAFLD however it is not essential. Insulin resistance is mediated by lipid accumulation, free fatty acids and altered mitochondrial metabolism. Adiponectine, Leptin derived from adipocytes modulate insulin signalling. Reduced adiponectine production plays a prominent role in NAFLD.

Clinical presentation: Patient may remain asymptomatic. Obesity is evident. Patient may have diabetes, hyperlipidemia. He may suffer from sleep apnea due to obesity. Hepatomegaly is present. Acanthosis nigricans is common. AST, ALT levels are raised.

INVESTIGATIONS

- Abnormal ALT, AST less than two times the normal has been reported. ALT/AST ratio less than one indicates mild disease while more than two indicates fibrosis.

- Blood sugar estimation, Hb A1C
- Serum lipid levels including abnormal lipoprotein profile
- Insulin resistance test
  - HOMA: Homeostasis model assessment
  - QUICKI test: Quantitative insulin sensitivity check test
- Hyperuricemia is common and thought to result from abnormal ATP metabolism
- Serum IgA levels are mildly elevated reflecting oxidative injury
- Abnormal iron indices are seen in 20–60% of cases, in severe cases ferritin is markedly elevated
- 30% of NASH patients have anti-nuclear antibodies.

Liver Imaging

Conventional imaging like sonography, CT scan is insensitive when hepatic fat content is less than 20% by weight. Secondly, it is unable to grade NASH.

Ultrasonography of a fatty liver shows a bright echotexure with heterogenous appearance. Ultrasonic elastography gives a measure of hepatic fibrosis. If BMI is >30 kg/m² may pose difficulty in obtaining signal.

Unenhanced CT scan of the fatty liver shows hypodense liver compared to the spleen. A liver/spleen ratio in Hounsfield unit of less than one is consistent with steatosis. Visceral versus peripheral fat distribution can be assessed by determining fat at a specific level such as L4–L5 cross-sectional imaging.

MRI is insensitive in detecting steatohepatitis but MR spectroscopy provides quantitative estimates of triglyceride content.

Liver Biopsy

It is the standard for confirming diagnosis, staging, grading activity and monitoring response to therapy. Being invasive, it is defered till the primary treatment of diet and exercise fails to give desired response. Biopsy may be problematic in obese individual.

Various parameters are combined in

NAI: NASH activity index and

NAS: NAFLD activity score

NAI ranges from 0 to 12. It accounts for steatosis, necroinflammation, hepatocyte injury, each of which is scored separately from 0–4.

NAS: Scale varies from 0–8.

Steatosis 0–3

Lobular/portal inflammation 0–3

Cellular ballooning 0–2

Secondary NASH

- Drug induced steatohepatitis—Number of drugs have been reported to cause steatosis. Many of them also lead to redistribution of body fat. This is known as lipodystrophy.
- Solvents and Industrial toxins—They are implicated in steatosis. These forms have also been known as TASH (toxicant associated steatohepatitis)
- Macro-and micro-vesicular steatosis is a potentially severe side effect of total parenteral nutrition.
- Severe protein malnutrition also can be associated with steatosis due to decreased apolipoprotein B.
- Celiac disease is seen in 3–4% of NASH cases even in the absence of weight loss.

- Wilson and other inherited metabolic diseases are associated with fatty liver though the mechanism are not well-understood.

MANAGEMENT

As yet there is no consensus on the definition, the bio-markers are not defined, the time duration for the progression of steatosis to cirrhosis or HCC is uncertain therefore the therapeutic end points remain ill-defined. Many molecules are being developed and some are under trial but RCTs-randomised controlled trials are lacking.

The management can be considered as:

1. Dietary modification/modification of lifestyle
2. Bariatric surgery
3. Pharmacotherapy
4. Liver transplant

1. Lifestyle modification

Lifestyle intervention: Counselling and perpetual motivation are essential. Diet modification based on ideal body weight and fat intake <30% of daily calories along with regular exercise can be accomplished in obese patients with success as high as 80% in achieving dietary goals and about 36% achieving exercise goal. Successful intervention can significantly reduce liver fat. Nutritional counselling with weight reduction is associated with improved aminotransferases and is in parallel with improved insulin signaling. It results in histological improvement.

Fast food needs to be avoided. It has been shown in healthy volunteers that fastfood-based hyper-alimentation can induce rapid and profound elevation in serum alanine aminotransferase.

Concentrated fructose sweeteners in soft drinks induce fatty liver in absence of metabolic syndrome. There is an evidence showing that it may lead to greater fibrosis. It should be avoided. Studies reveal fructose to be steatogenic.

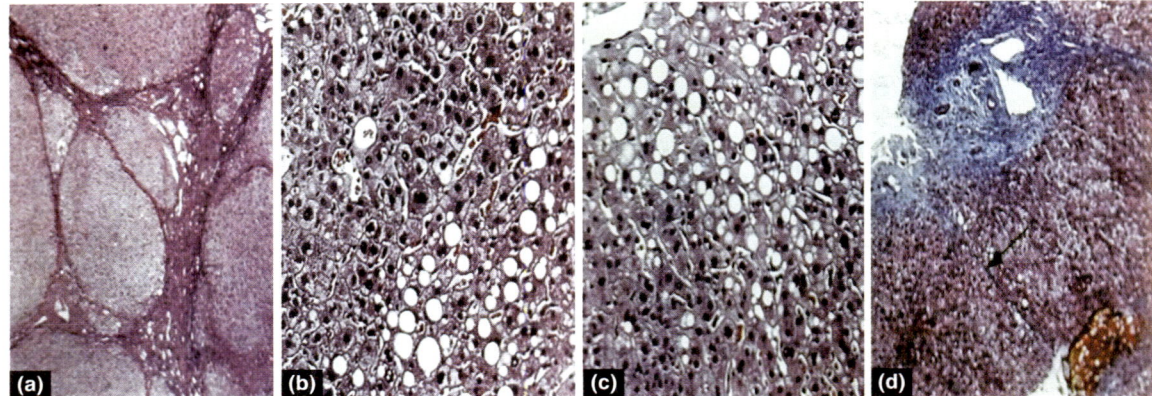

Fig.13.2: These pictures are from a obese diabetic person who underwent liver transplant for cryptogenic cirrhosis. Figure (a) shows explanted cirrhotic liver. Two years after transplant, patient had abnormal liver enzymes hence liver biopsy was done which revealed steatosis. (b) A year later biopsy showed persistent steatosis with inflammation. (c) Four years after transplant patient developed ascites, biopsy showing cirrhosis (d).

Diet adjuncts: Antioxidents like vitamin E 1000 mg/day and vitamin C 1000 mg/day decrease oxidative stress, improve aminotransferase level, have shown improvement in fibrosis in limited studies but has no action on inflammation and necrosis.

Suppliments with omega 3 fatty acid are not yet substantiated.

Weight loss agents

Orlistat: (Tetrahydrolipostatin)

It inhibits lipase thereby decreases fat absorption. Pilot studies were promising but RCTs showed similar weight loss in control and study group.

2. Bariatric surgery

Weight reduction surgery is indicated after failure of conventional weight loss programme. It is indicated if BMI is >40 kg/m² or >35 kg/m² in case of co-morbidities. Currently steatohepatitis is not considered as comorbidity. It has little effect on fibrosis.

3. Pharmacotherapy

Lipid lowering agents—No effect on inflammation or fibrosis have been documented.

Losartan—Angitensin 2 is shown to play a role in liver fibrosis, losartan has shown beneficial effects on sero-markers of fibrosis.

Metformin—It increases fatty acid oxidation in adipocytes but has no effect on NASH.

Thiozolidinediones—TZDs-pioglitazone Several trials have shown consistant improvement in aminotranferases, reduced hepatic steatosis, improved insulin siganalling but very little effect on fibrosis. In fact, weight gain was seen in large number of patients.

4. Liver Transplant

NASH/NAFLD are increasingly becoming designated indications for liver transplant. It has been shown that if lifestyle modification has failed to control obesity prior to surgery, the transplanted liver may also develop NAFLD (Fig. 13.2).

Lifestyle intervention with maintenance of normal weight is necessary to prevent NAFLD. It is running a parallel epidemic with obesity and diabetes.

14

Liver in Pregnancy

Alaka Deshpande

When an adult female conceives, she is known as a pregnant mother. During pregnancy there are changes in mother's physiology. Body metabolism is altered, nutritional requirements change. One has to think of mother and the foetus. The mother, the pregnancy outcome, the foetus/newborn are the most important considerations of a clinician.

The pre-conception counselling of the prospective parents is necessary. There has to be pregnancy preparedness. The pre-existing ailments need to be cared for. Necessary vaccinations may be given.

Normal pregnancy may show
- Palmer erythema, vascular spiders
- Decreased
  - Hematocrit, albumin
  - Bilirubin
  - Gamma: GT
- Increased alkaline phosphatase is generated by placenta and bone isoenzymes.

The liver diseases in pregnancy can be classified as:
- Pre-existing, e.g. HBV, autoimmune hepatitis
- Co-incidental, e.g. viral hepatitis HAV, HEV
- Specific to pregnancy
  - Acute fatty liver of pregnancy
  - HELLP syndrome
  - Intrahepatic cholestasis

Co-incidental infections can be viral hepatitis
- HAV, HEV, HBV, HCV
  - HSV2, CMV,
  - EBV, coxsackie
- Malaria.

Following drug therapy may affect liver functions as in non-pregnant women.
- ATT, ART
- Aldomet
- Valproic acid
- Steroids
- Amoxy—clavulanic acid
- Chlorpromazine

Viral Hepatitis

HAV and HEV are both transmitted by faeco-oral route. The infections are common in countries where awareness about personal hyegine is poor. The sewerage system is inadequate, contamination of drinking water spreads the infection.

In India, hepatitis A is an uncommon cause of acute viral hepatitis in pregnancy as most of the women in their early years have had overt or subclinical infection resulting into development of protective antibody. However, sporadic cases can occur in persons unexposed in childhood. HAV has no known effects on the foetus. In endemic regions, HAV vaccination should be a part of pre-conception counselling.

Viral Hepatitis HAV

- HAV, feco-oral route, epidemic any trimester
- Anorexia vomiting, pain RHC, high colored urine
- SGOT, SGPT↑ bilirubin↑
- Viral markers
  Anti HAV Ig M—Positive
- High-risk exposure of mother—Immunoprophylaxis
  Anti-HAV IgG 0.02 mg/kg within 2 weeks of exposure
- HAV in third trimester immunoprophylaxis to infant in 48 hr.
- Breastfeeding not contraindicated.

A pregnant mother who is at a high-risk of exposure should be protected by specific immunoglobulins which have been shown to be safe during pregnancy. HAV infection is not a contraindication to breastfeeding.

Viral Hepatitis E

Epidemic outbreaks of HEV are known. The infection is usually self-limiting in non-pregnant women but HEV infection during second and particularly in third trimester is associated with complications including fulminant hepatic failure. Some studies have reported acute liver failure in 22% of pregnancy + HEV cases. Several factors play a role; most important being decreased cell-mediated immunity which is probably due to high levels of circulating steroids during pregnancy. Presence of Anti-HEV IgM is diagnostic of HEV infection however in 20% of cases it may be negative. In these cases HEV RNA measurement is necessary. The management is symptomatic. Acute liver failure necessitates intensive care management.

Viral Hepatitis B

HBV infection is transmitted parenterally by infected blood, and blood products, infected injection needles, and unprotected multipartner sex, and vertically from infected pregnant mother to the foetus.

Table 14.1 shows transmission rates:

Pre-conception counselling should screen the mother for HbsAg. If she is a recipient of HBV vaccine anti HBV antibodies may be measured. If person is HbsAg negative and she is not vaccinated she may be offered HBV vaccine.

HBV vertical transmission rate is increased to 90% if mother is both HbsAg and Hb e Ag positive.

- Hbs Ag +ve   10–20%
- Hbs Ag +ve + Hb e +ve   90%
- Under these circumstances, in addition to the treatment of the mother the new-born needs to be protected.
  HBIG for the new-born
  – 1–2 ml (200 units) im within first 24 hrs.
  – 0.5 ml im immediat. after birth in HBV + HIV co-infected cases
- HB Vaccine to be started within 12 hrs.
- Breast feeding permitted in vaccinated child.

The management of HBV infected mother is shown in the Table 14.2.

Table 14.1: Vertical transmission

- HBV   10–20%
- HCV   5%
- HCV + HIV   14–40%
- HIV   30%

Table 14.2: Hepatitis B

Clinical	Viral markers	ALT	Treatment
Acute infection	Hbs Ag + Ig M Anti-Hb c +	ALT >10 × N	Spontaneous recovery
HBeAg positive	HBV DNA >20,000	Raised ALT	Treat
HbeAg negative	HBV DNA >2000	Raised ALT	Treat
Inactive carrier	HBeAg neg and HBV DNA <2000	ALT Normal	No therapy
Vaccinated	HBsAb++	—	Protected from infection

Antivirals like lamivudin, tenofovir, entecavir and interferon are used.

HCV Infection

Patients infected with HCV usually present with subclinical infection but during pregnancy patient may present with acute hepatitis C. Positive anti-HCV test during pregnancy need to be confirmed with HCV RNA levels. RNA level <10^6 copies indicates low level of transmission. If the RNA levels are more than 10^6, the transmission risk is high. If a woman is detected to be HCV positive before pregnancy she should be treated fully before conception. During this period she should use contraception.

The anti-HCV drugs are not safe during pregnancy so either the treatment should be postponed till delivery counselling the patient regarding risk of perinatal transmission. If the treatment is to be started during pregnancy she should be counselled for therapeutic termination of pregnancy.

Pre-existing conditions like auto-immune hepatitis, patients should be advised contraception till the disease is fully under control. The treatment of AIH consists of steroids which are safe but other immuno-suppressants like azathioprine is known to cross the placenta and has been shown to be terratogenic in experimental animal.

The liver diseases specific to pregnancy are:

1. Intrahepatic cholestasis.
2. Acute fatty liver of pregnancy
3. HELLP syndrome.

Intrahepatic cholestasis. It is seen in third trimester of pregnancy. Patient may have a family history or a history of the same ailment in previous pregnancy. Woman presents with jaundice and pruritus. The itching may be severe. There is a risk of prematurity and stillbirth. The bilirubin is increased. Serum alkaline phosphatise is elevted. There is a mild rise in aminotransfearase. The treatment comprises of:

- Cholestyramine 10–12 gm for pruritus
- Ursodeoxycholic acid at doses 15–20 mg/kg/day reduces fetal mortality and pruritus.

Acute Fatty Liver of Pregnancy

Acute fatty liver of pregnancy is associated with one of the inherited defects of mitochondrial beta-oxidation of fatty acids, long chain 3-hydroxyacyl CoA dehydrogenase deficiency. The mother and her foetus may be having this inherited enzyme deficiency. This leads to micro-vesicular fatty infiltration of the hepatocytes. Early diagnosis and prompt delivery may improve the prognosis, delay may prove fatal.

The patient may present with anorexia, abdominal pain. Pre-eclampsia may be associated. Aminotransferases are elevated but <500 IU, serum bilirubin is raised so also uric acid, creatinine and hypoglycaemia. Coagulation profile is deranged. Ultrasonography reveals fatty liver. Liver biopsy is diagnostic shows steatosis with fatty infiltration. However, it is not routinely required.

Swansea criteria for AFLP

- Vomiting
- Abdominal pain
- Polyuria/polydipsia
- Encephalopathy
- Bilirubin >14 µmol/L
- Urea >340 µmol/L
- Hypoglycaemia <4 µmol/L
- Leukocytosis 11 × 10^3/L
- ALT > 42 IU/L
- S. Ammonia >47 µmol/L
- Creatinine >150 µmol/L
- PT >14 seconds and APTT >34 seconds
- Biopsy
- Microvesicular steatosis

LIVER AND PREGNANCY (Table 14.3)

It is characterised by haemolysis with micro-angiopathic blood smear, elevated liver enzymes, and low platelet count. It is a severe

Table 14.3: Effects on liver during pregnancy

Diagnosis	Intra-hepatic cholestasis	Acute fatty liver of pregnancy	Acute viral hepatitis	HELLP syndrome
% Pregnancies	0.1 (USA)	0.005–0.01%	HEV more common in pregnancy	0.2–0.6%
Onset/Trimester	25–32 weeks	3 rd trimester or postpartum	Any	Third trimester or postpartum
Family history	Often	Occasionally	In epidemics	No
Presence of pre-eclampsia	No	50%	—	Yes
Salient clinical features	Pruritus	Liver failure with coagulopathy, encephalopathy	Prodrome	Abdominal pain
Presenting symptoms	Pruritus	Nausea, vomiting	Anorexia	Upper abdominal pain
Bilirubin	<5 mg %	Variable	Variable	<5 mg %
SGOT	<300 IU/L	<500 IU/L	<500 IU/L	<500 IU/L
Alk phos	Raised >4 folds ULN	Variable	Variable	Variable
Prothrombin time	May be prolonged, correctible with vitamin K	May be prolonged	May be prolonged	May be prolonged
Platelets	Usually normal	Thrmbocytopenia possible	Low in fulminant cases	< 100,000/cmm
Viral markers	Negative	Negative	Positive	Negative
Sonography	Normal	Normal, or smaller liver	Normal or hepatomegaly	Normal or enlarged liver
Additional features	Family or prior personal H/O IHCP	Non-specific symptoms followed by jaundice in 1–2 wk, if untreated FHF	—	Prior pre-eclamsia, eclampsia, micro-angiopathic haemolytic anaemia
Liver biopsy when permissible	Cholestasis with minimal or no inflammation	Micro-vesicular fatty infiltration	Widespread inflammation	Periportal haemmorhagic necrosis, fibrin deposition

HELLP Syndrome

- Hemolysis with microangiopathic blood smear
- ELevated liver enzymes
- LP low platelet count
- Severe variant of pre-eclampsia
- Abnormal placentation with complement mediated inflammation

variant of pre-eclampsia but the correlation between these two conditions is poorly understood. Most likely pathogenetic mechanism is abnormal placentation with complement mediated inflammation.

Signs and symptoms develop commonly between 28 and 36 weeks of gestation, but second trimester or postpartum onset is not uncommon. Patient presents with non-specific symptoms like epigastric pain, nausea, vomiting. Most patients (more than 85% cases) have hypertension and proteinuria.

Tennessee classification requires the presence of all of the following criteria to diagnose HELLP:

- Microangiopathic haemolytic anaemia with characteristic schistocytes (also called helmet cells) on blood smear. Other signs suggestive of haemolysis include an elevated indirect bilirubin level and a low serum haptoglobin concentration (≤25 mg/dL).
- Platelet count ≤100,000 cells/µL
- Total bilirubin ≥1.2 mg/dL (20.52 µmol/L)
- Serum AST ≥70 IU/L.

Mississippi classification is widely used to define HELLP syndrome as:

- Haemolysis documented by an increased LDH level and progressive anaemia
- Hepatic dysfunction documented by an LDH level >600 IU/L, elevated liver enzymes documented by AST >40 IU/L, AST >40 IU/L, or both
- Thrombocytopenia documented by a platelet nadir less than 1,50,000 cells/mm³. Thrombocytopenia is subclassified as class one HELLP syndrome: platelet nadir ≤50,000 cells/mm³, class two HELLP syndrome: platelet nadir ≤1,00,000 cells/mm³, or class three HELLP syndrome: platelet nadir ≤1,50,000 (Fig. 14.1).

Management

1. Stabilize the mother
2. Assess the foetal condition

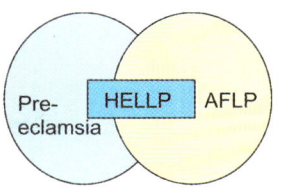

Fig. 14.1: HELLP syndrome

3. Antihypertensive drugs-labetalol, hydralazine, nifedipine, Na nitroprusside if severe hypertension.
4. Magnesium sulphate IV to prevent convulsions
5. Platelet transfusion if platelets <20,000, or e/o bleeding
6. Decision for prompt delivery
7. Liver transplant

In summary

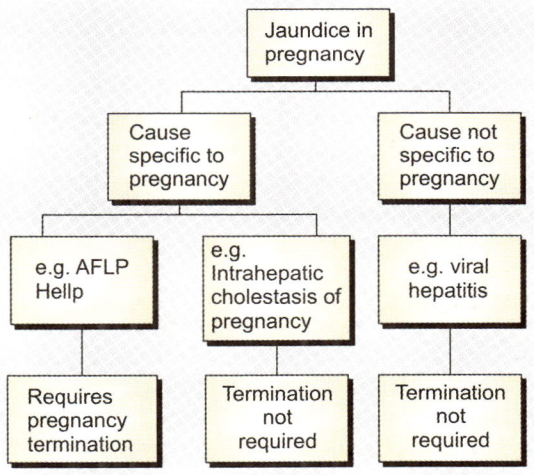

15

Liver Neoplasms

Alaka Deshpande

Benign focal lesions of the liver are increasingly being identified with advances in imaging technology. They can be benign neoplasms arising from the hepatocytes, supporting mesenchymal tissues or epithelium of the bile ducts (Table 15.1). Most of the benign tumours of the liver remain asymptomatic. Rarely complications like haemorrhage, rupture can occur.

In addition, there can be focal nodular hyperplasia, nodular regenerative hyperplasia or polycystic disease of the liver.

MALIGNANCY OF HEPATOCELLULAR CARCINOMA (HCC)

Primary liver cancer is the sixth most common cancer in the world and third cause of cancer related mortality. There are geographic variations mostly related to the prevalence of HBV and HCV and the availability of HBV immunization. Gender, geographic area, risk factors associated with cancer determine the age at which HCC appears (Table 15.2).

RISK FACTORS FOR HCC

Cirrhosis underlies the HCC in more than 80% of cases. Any agent causing chronic liver damage and ultimately leading to cirrhosis should be considered as a risk factor.

Pathogenesis

The molecular mechanisms are not yet known but oxidative damage with active inflammation is thought to be leading to cancer.

In viral hepatitis, repeated episodes of inflammation and regeneration result in increased rate of DNA mutation. Probably the DNA repair rate is decreased. Accumulation of mutated DNA leads to development of HCC.

Table 15.1: Benign tumours of the liver

- Epithelial tumours
  - Hepatocellular adenoma
  - Bile duct adenoma
  - Biliary papillomatosis
- Mesenchymal tumours
  - Hemangioma
  - Fibroma
  - Lipoma
  - Lymphangioma
  - Angiomyolipoma
  - Hamartoma

Table 15.2: Liver diseases associated with HCC

Cirrhotic	Non-cirrhotic
Hepatitis B	Hepatitis B
Hepatitis C	Hepatitis C
Alcoholic cirrhosis	Hepatic adenoma
NAFLD	
Autoimmune hepatitis	
Primary biliary cirrhosis	
Hemochromatosis	
Alpha-antitrypsin deficiency	

Pathology

HCC develops over several years. The changes occur at a genetic level without morphological changes.

Pathological appearance depends upon the stage of malignancy from early to advanced stage. The pathological changes may be described as expansive:

Gross appearance showing a distinct margin and a reticulin pseudocapsule may be described as expansive nodule. Infiltrative type does not show distinct margins. Diffuse type mimics a cirrhotic liver, it is multinodular tumour, 30–40% of tumours show fat deposition.

Immunostaining can identify many proteins such as alpha-fetoprotein (AFP), carcino-embryonic antigen (CEA) and cytokeratins like 7, 8, 18, 19. However, the usual biomarkers like alpha-fetoprotein, glycosylated AFP, des gamma carboxy prothrombin are not expressed in early HCC.

Clinical Presentation

HCC appears in the setting of cirrhosis therefore, clinical picture is mostly of the advanced cirrhosis. Patient may present with jaundice, ascites, hepatic encephalopathy or with signs and symptoms of portal hypertension. Imaging and tumour markers help in diagnosis.

If the patient presents with constitutional symptoms of malignancy like weight loss, anorexia, abdominal pain, the cancer may be in the advanced stages and cure may be unlikely.

Rarely patient may present with bone metastasis. There are reports of patient presenting with haemoperitoneum due to ruptured HCC.

HCC has the distinction of presenting with paraneoplastic syndrome. Patient may present with frequent hypoglycaemia due to raised production of insulin like peptide, hypercalcaemia, venous thrombosis due to hypercoagulable state. When a case of liver disease presents with such symptoms he may be subjected to abdominal sonography and tumour marker studies are indicated.

If AFP is greater than 200 ng/ml in a case having mass in the liver, the possibility of HCC is greater than 90% and biopsy is not required.

Surveillance for HCC

Early detection of HCC is possible by regular screening of at risk patients by sonography and estimation of α-feto proteins. The known risk factors are HBV, HCV infections, cirrhosis.

- Investigations
- Liver function tests,
- HbsAg, anti-HCV antibodies
- Abdominal sonography
- α-fetoproteins
- CT scan brain

Prognostication

Prognostication should take into consideration liver functions, tumour mass, and nodes, metastasis. Various scoring systems exist but Barcelona clinic liver cancer (BCLC) system considers all evolving systems and is well-validated.

Management

Large number of therapeutic techniques are available

- Liver resection
- Liver transplantation
- Hepatic artery ligation
- Hepatic artery embolization
- Chemo-embolization
- Internal radiotherapy
- External beam radiotherapy
- Chemotherapy
- Local ablation
  a. Radiofrequency ablation
  b. Cryotherapy
- Targated agents

Resection—About 40% HCC cases in Asia and 5% cases in western countries which are without cirrhosis; resection of the liver is the treatment of choice. These cases tolerate major resections with a very low-risk of morbidity.

Transplantation—It provides excellent outcomes if restricted to patients in early stages of the disease defined by Milano criteria:

- Solitary nodule <5 cm.
- Up to three nodules each measuring <3 cm.

Survival exceeds more than 70% at 5 yrs.

Hepatic artery ligation/embolization/chemoembolization. In most of the cases HCC receives blood supply from the hepatic artery. Blockage of the hepatic artery results into tumour ischaemia and necrosis.

Chemotherapy—Systemic chemotherapies have only marginal effect. Understanding of the molecular pathways of tumour proliferation it has been shown that inhibition of angiogenesis can have anti-tumour activity. VEGF inhibitor—Sorafenib is the drug which is given orally. It is a multikinase inhibitor which acts by blocking the different signalling pathways associated with hepatocarcinogenesis. The limitations are its serious side-effects.

The other therapies did not show survival benefit over untreated patients.

16

Liver Transplantation

Somnath Chattopadhyay,
Upasna Bahure, Ravi Mohanka, Samir Shah

Liver transplant is the procedure of replacing a severely damaged cirrhotic, failing or dysfunctional liver with a functionally normal one. Initial attempts at transplantation were met with failure secondary to profound technical difficulties, severe bleeding, high complication rates, high graft failure rates and mortality. It has subsequently evolved into a safe operation and is presently the standard of care for treatment of cirrhosis with end-stage liver disease (ESLD), acute liver failure (ALF) and hepatocellular cancer (HCC).

The West took the lead in defining the legal framework, logistic support and infrastructure required for retrieval of solid organs from brain dead donors and developed deceased donor liver transplantation (DDLT). While this led to an increase in the number of transplants in most western countries, it was soon realized that the demand for liver transplant was far more than the availability of donor organs. Living donor liver transplant (LDLT) was one of the ways to fill this gap. This gap was more obvious in some Eastern countries such as India, Korea, and Japan where organ donation rates were very low; probably because of differences in socio-cultural beliefs, public awareness, health care, economic structure and availability of expertise. Necessitated by the situation, centres in these Asian countries embarked on LDLT programs and in the process gained a large experience and pioneered several surgical techniques in LDLT. Currently while in the west, most liver transplants performed are DDLT, while in the East, LDLT is predominant.

Aetiologies, Indications and Organ Allocation for Liver Transplant

An outline of aetiology for liver failure and indications for liver transplant is given in Tables 16.1 and 16.2 and further discussed below.

Cirrhosis with chronic end stage liver disease (ESLD). Viral hepatitis due to hepatitis B (HBV) and C (HCV) are the most common aetiologies of ESLD requiring transplant, about 20–25% each, although there are huge regional variations. With widely implemented vaccination programs for HBV, routine screening programmes in blood banks and effective anti-viral drugs for both HBV and HCV (directly acting antivirals), both these are on a decline and are expected to become less important indications for transplant in the future. On the other hand, alcoholic and non-alcoholic fatty liver disease leading to ESLD are increasing and assuming significant proportions. Other diseases like auto-immune hepatitis (AIH), drug induced liver injury (DILI), primary sclerosing cholangitis (PSC) and primary

Table 16.1: Aetiology and indications for liver transplant	
Aetiology-adults	*Aetiology-children*

Chronic Liver Disease

• Viral (hepatitis B or C)	• Biliary atresia (BA) (most common)
• Alcoholic	• Alagille's syndrome
• Non-alcoholic steatohepatitis (NASH)/non-alcoholic fatty liver disease (NAFLD)	• Non-syndromic biliary hypoplasia
	• Familial intrahepatic cholestasis
• Cryptogenic	• Auto-immune hepatitis
• Auto-immune hepatitis (AIH)	• Viral (hepatitis B, C, other)
• Drug-induced liver injury (DILI) (Anti-TB/ Ayurvedic/ratol/dapsone/others)	• Cryptogenic
• Primary biliary cirrhosis (PBC)	
• Primary sclerosing cholangitis (PSC)	
• Cystic fibrosis (CF)	

Liver Tumours

• Hepatocellular carcinoma (HCC)	• Hepatoblastoma
• Benign tumours (rarely)	• HCC (uncommon)
• Other tumours (metastatic neuroendocrine tumours)	• Benign tumours (rarely)

Acute Liver Failure

• Fulminant to subacute viral hepatitis (A, B or E)	• Autoimmune
• AIH related liver failure	• Toxin (Halothane/Paracetamol)
• Toxin-drugs (Paracetamol)	• Viral hepatitis (A, B, C, E or NA-G)
• Pregnancy related	• Indeterminate
• Amanita poisoning	
• Wilson's disease	
• Indeterminate	
• α1-antitrypsin deficiency (A1A)	
• Haemochromatosis	
• Wilson's disease	

Metabolic Diseases

• Budd-Chiari syndrome	• α1-antitrypsin deficiency
• Polycystic liver disease	• Cystic fibrosis
• Amyloidosis	• Glycogen storage disease (type IV)
• Non-cirrhotic portal fibrosis	• Tyrosinemia (type I)
	• Wilson's disease
	• Crigler-Najjar (type I)
	• Familial hypercholesterolemia
	• Fatty acid oxidation defects
	• Primary oxalosis
	• Organic acidemia
	• Urea cycle defects
	• Fibropolycystic liver disease

Others

Table 16.2: Disease severity assessment in cirrhosis with end-stage liver disease (ESLD)

Child-Turcotte-Pugh (CTP) score

Points	1	2	3
Serum total bilirubin [µmol/L (mg/dL)]	<34 (< 2)	34–50 (2–3)	>50 (> 3)
Serum albumin (g/L)	>35	28–35	<28
Prothrombin time (INR)	<1.7	1.71–2.2	>2.2
Ascites	None	Controlled with diuretics	Refractory
Hepatic encephalopathy	None	Grade I–II	Grade III–IV

Prognostic implications of CTP score

Class	Score	Survival
A	5–6	90% at 5 years
B	7–9	80% at 5 years
C	10–15	60% at 1 year

MELD/PELD score and its variations

- MELD score (for patients > 12 years of age) = $9.57 \times \log$ [serum creatinine (mg/dL)] + $3.78 \times \log$ [serum bilirubin (mg/dL)] + $11.2 \times \log$ (INR) + 6.43 values range (6–40).
- MELD-Na = $9.57 \times \log$ [serum creatinine (mg/dL)] + $3.78 \times \log$ [serum bilirubin (mg/dL)] + $11.2 \times \log$ (INR) + 6.43 + $1.59 \times$ [135-serum sodium (mg/dL)].
- UKELD = $1.485 \times \log$ [serum creatinine (µmol/L)]) + $3.13 \times \log$ [serum bilirubin (µmol/L)] + $5.395 \times \log$ (INR) + $81.565 \times \log$ [serum sodium (mmol/L)] + 435.
- PELD score (patients up to 12 years) = $0.480 \times \log$ [serum bilirubin (mg/dL)] + $1.857 \times \log$ (INR) $-0.687 \times \log$ [serum albumin (g/dL)] + 0.436 (if the patient is < 1 year old) + 0.667 [if the patient has growth failure (≤ 2 standard deviation)].

Prognostic implications of MELD score

MELD score	3 month survival (%)	1 year survival (%)
0–998	90	
10–19	94	80
20–29	81	66
30–35	48	33
> 35	29	

Indications for liver transplant based on complications of ESLD

Complication
- Refractory ascites
- Refractory portal hype rtensive haemorrhage (variceal bleed)
- Spontaneous bacterial peritonitis (SBP)
- Recurrent hepatic encephalopathy
- Hepato-renal syndrome
- Hepato-pulmonary syndrome
- Biliary cirrhosis
- Diuretic-induced nephropathy
- Portal vein thrombosis
- Compromised quality of life
- Growth retardation or failure to thrive in children

(Contd.)

Table 16.2: Disease severity assessment in cirrhosis with end-stage liver disease (ESLD) *(Contd.)*

Aetiology-specific scoring systems

Alcoholic liver disease
- Maddrey (modified) DF calculated as = 4.6 × (prolongation of prothrombin time in seconds) + serum bilirubin (mg/dL). A modified DF score > 32 in the presence of hepatic encephalopathy predicts >50% mortality within 28 days in patients with alcoholic hepatitis.
- GAHS (2005): GAHS is a composite scoring system based on age, serum bilirubin, blood urea nitrogen, prothrombin time and the peripheral leukocyte count. GAHS ≥9 is a predictor of mortality and is more accurate than DF in predicting both 28- and 84-day mortality.
- Lille model incorporates age, renal insufficiency, albumin, prothrombin time, bilirubin and the evolution of bilirubin on day 7 to predict 6-month mortality in patients with severe alcoholic hepatitis who have received corticosteroid therapy.

Primary sclerosing cholangitis (PSC)
- Mayo PSC risk score: R = 0.03 × (age in years) + 0.54 × log (bilirubin in mg/dL) + 0.54 × log (AST in IU/L) + 1.24 × (history of variceal bleeding) – 0.84 × (albumin in g/dL).
- Primary biliary cirrhosis (PBC).
- Mayo risk score (R): 0.871 × log (bilirubin in mg/dL) – 2.53 × log (albumin in g/dL) + 0.039 × (age in years) + log × (prothrombin time in seconds) + 0:859 (if oedema is present).

Wilson's disease
- Nazer score: Based on serum bilirubin, AST and prothrombin time (each parameter graded on a 0–4 scale); cut-off > 7.
- New Wilson's index (revised Wilson's disease prediction index): Based on a combination of AST, albumin, bilirubin, INR and white cell count (each parameter was graded on a 0–4 scale); cut-off > 11.

Abbreviations: INR, international normalized ratio; MELD, model for end-stage liver disease; UKELD, United Kingdom model for end-stage liver disease; PELD, pediatric end-stage liver disease, CTP, Child-Turcotte-Pugh; CLD, chronic liver disease, DF, discriminant function; GAHS, Glasgow alcoholic hepatitis score; PSC, primary sclerosing cholangitis; AST, aspartate aminotransferase; INR, international normalized ratio.

Biliary cirrhosis (PBC) are less common but important indications for liver transplant. In about 15–20% of patients, the cause cannot be ascertained and they are termed as cryptogenic.

Assessment of disease severity and prognostication is done using various scoring systems, commonly used being Child-Turcotte-Pugh (CTP) grade and model for end stage liver disease (MELD) score. In certain situations, these scores may not truly reflect disease severity, when alternative scoring systems or disease specific scoring systems are used for prognostication. ESLD patients with CTP grade C and MELD score > 14 are candidates for a transplant. Certain complications of ESLD, although increase the morbidity and mortality risk, may not reflect in disease severity scores (Table 16.2).

Organ Allocation Systems Based on Severity of Chronic Liver Disease

Unfortunately, all patients needing a transplant, based on these criteria are unable to have one because of shortage of livers from deceased donors. Therefore, most countries have an organ allocation system in place based on ethical principles of beneficence, equality, utility, justice and transparency. The criteria used for selection and mechanism of distribution of livers for DDLT differ between countries. While in some countries, the allocation is sequential based on the duration on the waiting list, in others it is based on disease severity, with sickest patients being offered the organ. Often, prioritization for local, regional or national patients and for multi-organ transplants is given. In USA, MELD score is used for prioritization and organ allocation, in Europe, allocation in various geographical areas is governed by different organ exchange organizations and protocols, e.g. United Kingdom Transplant (UKT), Eurotransplant, Scandiatransplant and others. In India, allocation of liver for DDLT varies in each state. In most allocation systems, a provision for giving exceptional priority to certain cases based on peer review is built-in, for situations where the disease severity is not truly reflected in the score used. Despite all efforts to increase the number of organ donations, the number of organ donations has only been modest while patients continue to face a high waiting list mortality risk.

Hepatocellular Cancer (HCC)

Liver transplantation is the best option for patients with cirrhosis and HCC, because not only it offers complete resection with the widest surgical margin (total hepatectomy), it also eliminates the potentially tumorigenic environment of cirrhotic liver. HCC contributes about 10–25% of transplants. Until the 1990s, patients with advanced HCC had very high recurrence rates and poor survival after liver transplant. However, when liver transplant was offered only to patients with small HCC, very good outcomes were achieved. Patients with HCC typically have low liver disease severity scores, very long waiting times on DDLT and therefore are at a disadvantage on the waiting list and also carry a definite risk of tumour progression.

Organ Allocation for HCC Patients

In the United States, patients with HCC within the Milan criteria (based on tumour size and number) are given MELD exception points to prioritize them on the waiting list. This gives HCC patients a fair chance at transplant and has led to good outcomes. Similar prioritization criteria are used in most allocation systems. With improved imaging and availability of multimodality treatments including transarterial chemoembolization (TACE),

radiofrequency ablation (RFA), and transarterial radio-embolization (TARE), excellent outcomes can now be achieved.

LDLT inherently has a shorter waiting time, which in turn reduces the risk of tumour progression. Most centres now find Milan criteria to be too restrictive and use the University of California San Francisco (UCSF) or other more liberal criteria, which are not uniform across the world (Table 16.3).While use of more liberal criteria allows more HCC patients to undergo transplant, they carry a higher risk of recurrence, this is also called as the "Metro Ticket Concept" (Fig. 16.1).

Acute Liver Failure (ALF)/Fulminant Hepatic Failure (FHF)

Acute liver failure is a rare but critical illness characterized by rapid deterioration of liver functions and development of encephalopathy usually in the absence of pre-existing liver disease. Hepatic dysfunction is in the form of jaundice, coagulopathy, rising liver enzymes and development of hepatic encephalopathy. Fulminant hepatic failure was originally defined as development of encephalopathy within 8 weeks of onset of liver dysfunction. The time interval between development of liver dysfunction to encephalopathy provides clues to cause of liver failure and prognosis. 3–10% of transplants are for acute liver failure and the aetiology differs amongst age groups and geographically regions across the world. The most common aetiology of ALF among adults in the US and Europe is viral hepatitis (hepatitis A, B, E) while that in the UK is acetaminophen overdose related drug-induced liver injury (DILI). Metabolic diseases such as congenital hemochromatosis, galactosemia, tyrosinemia and mitochondrial cytopathies present early in children, while Wilson's disease generally presents later in childhood. In India, major causes of ALF are viral hepatitis (90%, hepatitis E > A > B) and DILI (anti-tuberculosis drugs and herbal preparations). About 15–20% cases are due to indeterminate cause.

Table 16.3: Various criteria for liver transplantation in HCC

Criteria	Single lesion (cm)	Multiple lesions No.	Size (cm)	Non-size criteria
Commonly used				
Milan	≤5	3	3	
UCSF	≤6.5	3	4.5	Sum of all diameters ≤8.5 cm
Other criteria				
Pittsburgh	Modified TNM staging			
Barcelona	<7	3	<5	
		5	<3	
Kyoto		≤ 10	≤5	PIVKA ≤400 mAU/mL
Hong Kong	≤6.5	3	≤4.5	
Tokyo (5–5 rule)		5	≤5	
Kneteman, Canada	<7.5	Any	<5	
Fukuoka, Japan		Any	Any	No gross vascular invasion or extra-hepatic spread
Hangzhou criteria	≤8 cm			
	>8 cm			Grade I or II and AFP ≤400
New Milan (up to 7)	Sum of number of tumours + diameter of largest tumour ≤7			
Edmonton	Total tumour volume ≤115 mL, AFP ≤400 ng/mL			
Asan criteria		≤6	≤5	No gross vascular invasion

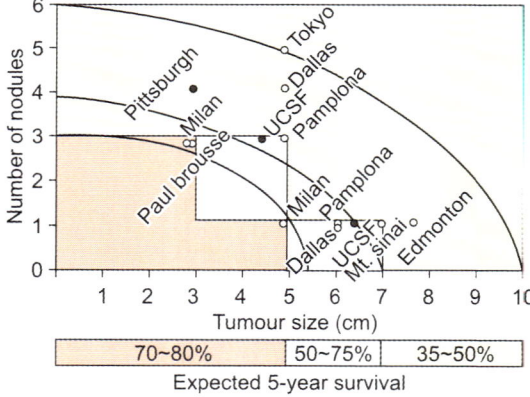

Fig. 16.1: Beyond Milan criteria-HCC 'Metro ticket', the further the distance, the higher the price

King's College Criteria (KCC) is the most widely used criteria to assess the potential for spontaneous recovery in ALF patients and therefore the need for transplant. Patients meeting KCC are given the highest priority on the waiting list and allotted an organ out of turn for an emergency liver transplant. Other criteria like Villejuif-Clichy criteria, acute physiology and chronic health evaluation II (APACHE II) score, MELD score, hepatocyte necrosis on liver biopsy and diminishing liver volume on serial imaging are also used for prognostication (Table 16.4).

Acute on Chronic Liver Failure (ACLF)

Acute on chronic liver failure is a distinct entity involving acute deterioration of liver function in the presence of chronic liver disease. Asia-Pacific association for study of liver (APASL) defines ACLF as an acute hepatic insult manifesting as jaundice and coagulopathy, complicated within 4 weeks by ascites and/or encephalopathy in a patient with previously diagnosed or undiagnosed chronic liver disease. The American and the European study groups (AASLD and EASL), on the other hand, define ACLF as acute deterioration of pre-existing, chronic liver disease, usually related to a precipitating event and associated with increased mortality at 3 months due to multi-system organ failure.

Table 16.4: Disease severity assessment in acute liver failure

Criteria	Aetiology	Prognostic markers
King's College Criteria	Acetaminophen	• Arterial blood pH <7.30 (irrespective of grade of encephalopathy) Or all of the following: • Prothrombin time >100 seconds (INR >6.5) • Serum creatinine >300 µmol/L • Grade III/IV hepatic encephalopathy
King's College Criteria	Non-acetaminophen	• Prothrombin time >100 seconds (INR >6.5) irrespective of grade of encephalopathy Or any three of the following (irrespective of grade of encephalopathy) • Age <10 or >40 years • Aetiology: non-A/non-B hepatitis, drug-induced • Duration of jaundice to encephalopathy >7 days • Prothrombin time >50 seconds (INR >3.5) • Serum bilirubin >300 µmol/L
Clichy criteria	All	HE + factor V <20% (age <30 years) or <30% (age >30 years)
Factor V; factor VIII/V ratio	Acetaminophen	Factor VIII/V ratio > 30 Factor V < 10%
APACHE II	All	APACHE II >19
Gc-globulin	All	Gc-globulin <100 mg/L
Lactate	Acetaminophen	Admission arterial lactate >3.5 or >3.0 mmol/L after fluid resuscitation
AFP	Acetaminophen	AFP < 3.9 mcg/L 24 h post-peak ALT
MELD	• Acetaminophen • Non-acetaminophen	 MELD >33 at onset of HE
Liver biopsy		Hepatocyte necrosis

Abbreviations: AFP-Alpha fetoprotein, APACHE II–Acute physiology and chronic health evaluation, Gc–Globulin-Group specific complement, HE- hepatic encephalopathy.

Most commonly affects young males with active alcoholism on underlying alcohol related liver disease, infection or untreated HBV hepatitis. The underlying mechanism is an excessive systemic inflammatory response to a pathogen or non pathogenic stimulus. Patients with 3 or more organ failures including renal and cerebral (grade 3 or 4 HE) is associated with a very high (about 70%) mortality risk. Few patients are able to undergo a liver transplant, with limited success rates.

Indications in Children

In children, biliary atresia is the most common indication for transplant, a large majority of them requiring it after failure of Kasai's portoenterostomy. Hepatoblastoma is the most common pediatric liver tumour requiring transplant, HCC is commonly found in children with tyrosinemia. Pediatric end stage liver disease (PELD) score is commonly used for assessment of liver disease severity and for organ allocation for children younger than 12 years in USA, however graft size for the child is often taken into consideration for allocation.

Metabolic Liver Diseases

Liver-specific metabolic diseases can be divided into:

1. Diseases that lead to liver injury, with or without other organ involvement, such as alpha-1-antitrypsin deficiency, Wilson's disease, tyrosinaemia, familial cholestasis and cystic fibrosis.
2. Diseases due to a metabolic defect expressed solely or predominantly in the liver causing injury to other organ systems, such as the urea cycle disorders, Crigler-Najjar syndrome and hyperoxaluria.

Allocation of deceased donor organs for metabolic liver diseases is often made on a case to case basis or a living donor transplant is performed.

Contraindications for Liver Transplant

Contraindications for liver transplant are:

- Active, extra-hepatic uncontrolled, multi-drug resistant or refractory infection, systemic sepsis or septic shock, severe acute lung injury or severe multi-organ system failure.
- Severe cardiopulmonary or other co-morbid conditions.
- Active psychiatric illness or lack of psycho-social support, active alcohol or other substance abuse. Relative contraindications are repeated suicide attempts or psychological instability.
- Anticipated major technical difficulty, e.g. extensive portal- mesenteric venous thrombosis (PVT).
- In patients with HCC, extra-hepatic or macro-vascular tumour involvement are absolute contraindications for liver transplant.
- In patients with ALF, intracranial pressure (ICP) greater than 35 mm of Hg, cerebral perfusion pressure (CPP) less than 40 mm

of Hg for more than 2 hours, fixed and dilated pupils, poor transcranial Doppler signal or any other features of brain death.
- In patients with hepato-pulmonary syndrome (HPS), preoperative PaO_2 <50 mm Hg and shunt fraction >20%.

Recipient Pre-transplant Evaluation

Evaluation includes a detailed history including that of alcohol or drug abuse, blood transfusions, liver decompensation, previous abdominal surgeries and co-morbidities. A thorough physical examination includes examination for fever, icterus, pedal oedema, ascites, hepatic encephalopathy and other signs.

Patients undergo a detailed evaluation by a multidisciplinary team consisting of transplant surgeons, transplant hepatologists, cardiologist, pulmonologist, psychiatrist, nutritionist, transplant co-ordinator and social worker. The goal of evaluation is:

a. Establish the severity of liver disease, indication, urgency and fitness for a liver transplant.
b. Listing for a deceased donor liver transplant if no contraindications exist and counselling for a living donor liver transplant if indicated.
c. Management of decompensation of liver disease like ascites, recurrent hepatic encephalopathy, renal dysfunction and portal hypertension in order to optimize the patient.
d. Planning for bridging/downstaging therapy for hepatocellular carcinoma in the form of TACE, TARE, RFA, etc.
e. Establish a system of periodic follow-up while waiting for an organ offer to prevent further deterioration.

Evaluation includes a detailed history including that of alcohol or drug abuse, blood transfusions, liver decompensation, previous abdominal surgeries and co-morbidities. A thorough physical examination includes examination for fever, icterus, pedal oedema, ascites, hepatic encephalopathy and other signs.

Laboratory tests include complete haemogram, coagulation profile, liver and renal function tests. Hepatitis B and C serology positive patients need viral PCR testing and serology for other viral infections such as cytomegalovirus (CMV), Epstein-Barr virus (EBV), Herpes simplex virus (HSV) and others. Autoimmune antibody screen, iron and copper profile may help determine aetiology. In patients with portal vein thrombosis or Budd-Chiari syndrome, a detailed thrombophillia profile is done to determine need for post-operative anticoagulation. Microbiologic screen is done to rule out active infections which includes blood, urine and ascitic fluid cultures and screening for Methicillin resistant *Staphylococcus aureus* (MRSA), Vancomycin-resistant *Enterococcus* (VRE) and Carbapenem-resistant *Enterococcus* (CRE). Thyroid, lipid and diabetes profiles are done to evaluate endocrine status and for pre-operative optimization.

Detailed cardio-respiratory risk analysis and evaluation is done with electrocardiogram (ECG), stress echocardiography (ECHO), pulmonary function tests (PFT), arterial blood gas (ABG), and coronary or pulmonary imaging. Patients with pulmonary artery systolic pressures (PASP) >45 mm Hg are further evaluated for Porto-pulmonary hypertension (PPHTN) by right heart catheterization. Hypoxaemia (PaO_2 <70 mm Hg on ABG) may suggest hepato-pulmonary syndrome (HPS) and should be confirmed by bubble ECHO and Tc99 macro-aggregated albumin scan.

Ultrasound with Doppler, tri-phasic computed tomography (CT) scan or magnetic resonance imaging (MRI) is done to evaluate for liver mass and outline the anatomy and patency of liver vessels. Patients with HCC undergo positron-emission tomography (PET) or HRCT chest/bone scan to evaluate extent of its spread. Screening tumour markers and in women a mammogram and PAP smear is done to rule out common malignancies. Upper and lower gastrointestinal endoscopy is done to evaluate portal hypertension (PHT) and rule out GI malignancies.

Donor Evaluation and Preparation

Deceased (Brain Dead/Cadaveric) Donor Selection

An ideal liver donor would be younger than 50 years with no pre-existing liver disease, normal LFTs at the time of death, no systemic infections and haemodynamically stable with good tissue perfusion and oxygenation. However, often, livers from donors beyond these criteria are used for transplant. Such donors are called as or marginal/extended criteria donors and although livers from them have a higher risk of complications, the risk of mortality on waiting list justifies their use. Severely steatotic livers (macro-vesicular steatosis >60%) or prolonged cold ischaemia time (>12 hours) significantly increases the risk of primary non-function (PNF). Hepatitis B and C virus positive donor livers can be selectively used in patients with corresponding viral infection related liver disease.

Donation after cardiac death (DCD), i.e. non-heart beating donors (NHBD) have severe brain injury incompatible with recovery but do not meet brainstem death criteria. Such donors are stratified into four categories and two groups: uncontrolled (categories 1 and 2) and controlled (categories 3 and 4). The risks of PNF and post-transplant intrahepatic biliary strictures are major concerns in use of these grafts. Currently, organ donation from DCD donors is not practiced in India. Contra-indications for using livers from deceased donors and the risk of disease transmission is listed in Table 16.5.

Living Donor Evaluation

Living liver donors are patients' family members, generally between 18 to 50 years old of compatible blood group with a non-fatty

Table 16.5		
Ideal donor	*(ECD) Marginal/Extended criteria donor*	*Donation after cardiac death (DCD)*
• 50 years or younger • No hepatobiliary disease • Normal LFTs • No severe abdominal trauma/ systemic infection/cancer • Hemodynamic and respiratory stability (systolic blood pressure >100 mm Hg, CVP >5 cm H$_2$O) • None or low vasopressor support (dopamine <10 µg/ kg/min) • Urine output >50 mL/hr and normal creatinine	• Steatosis (>30%), necrosis, fibrosis • Old age (>65 years) • Prolonged CIT (>10 hrs) • High LFTs (bilirubin >2 mg%, AST/ALT >four times normal) • Reactive serology (HBsAg, HCVab, HBcAb) • Donor BMI (>35) • High vasopressor support • ICU stay (>5 days) • High serum sodium (>160) • Active infection: positive blood cultures with MDR bugs • Malignancy (low grade brain or skin)	Maastricht classification • Type 1: Brought dead • Type 2: Unsuccessful resuscitation • Type 3: Awaiting cardiac arrest • Type 4: Cardiac arrest after brainstem death

Contraindications for organ donation
- Primary intra-cerebral lymphoma
- All secondary intracerebral tumours
- Any active (that is, not in remission) cancer with evidence of spread outside affected organ (including lymph nodes) within 3 years of donation (however, localised prostate, thyroid, *in situ* cervical cancer and non-melanotic skin cancers are acceptable).
- Melanoma (except completely excised stage 1 cancers)
- Active (not in remission) haematological malignancy (myeloma, lymphoma, leukaemia)
- Definite, probable or possible case of human transmissible spongiform encephalopathy (TSE), including CJD and vCJD, individuals whose blood relatives have had familial CJD, other neurodegenerative diseases associated with infectious agents.
- TB: active and untreated
- HIV disease (but not HIV infection)
- Active uncontrolled sepsis

Abbreviations: ECD, extended criteria donor; LFTs, liver function tests; CVP, central venous pressure; CIT, cold ischaemia time; AST, aspartate aminotransferase; ALT, alanine transaminase; HBsAg, hepatitis B surface antigen; HCVab, hepatitis C virus antibody; HBcAb, hepatitis B core antibody; BMI, body mass index; MDR, multidrug resistant.

liver. Potential donors are counseled about the evaluation process and their willingness is confirmed. A detailed history and physical examination are done. Haematological, biochemical and serological work-up includes haemogram, liver and renal function tests and viral markers. Liver steatosis is estimated by using liver attenuation index (LAI) on non-contrast CT scan. Triple phase CT liver angiogram is used to study the vascular anatomy of the liver and calculate the sectoral volumes. This is utilized for the calculation of graft to recipient weight ratio (GRWR = Graft weight (gm)/recipient weight (gm) × 100) and estimation of future donor remnant volume (FLR = Remnant liver volume/total liver volume × 100). Most centres accept grafts more than 0.8% of recipient body weight (GRWR >0.8%) and the remnant liver volume should be more than 30% of the total liver volume. A liver biopsy may be required in donors with high BMI, LAI < +5 or abnormal

LFTs. A magnetic resonance cholangio-pancreatography (MRCP) outlines the biliary anatomy.

Cardiorespiratory evaluation is done by ECG, ECHO and PFT and risk analysis by cardiologist and pulmonologist. Invasive coronary or pulmonary imaging and carotid Doppler may be indicated in older donors with other risk factors. The donor also undergoes gynaecology, hepatology, psychiatric and anaesthesia evaluation.

Inadequate volumes, steatosis and comorbidities remain important reasons for rejection of donors. The problem of low graft volume may be managed by graft inflow modulation or use of dual lobes in the recipient, both of which do not increase the donor risk. Donor steatosis may be reduced by following a dedicated exercise and weight loss regimen. However, potential donors with inadequate estimated remnant or significant medical risks should not be accepted for donation.

Surgical Technique

Donor Operation

Liver recovery from deceased donor is shown in Fig. 16.2. The goal of organ recovery from a deceased donor is to remove the warm blood and perfuse the donated organs with cold perfusion solution [Histidine-tryptophan-ketoglutarate (HTK) or University of Wisconsin (UW) solution] at 4°C. The abdomen and chest are opened with a midline incision and sternotomy. A rapid exploration of the abdominal cavity is done to rule out tumours. Liver is grossly accessed for colour, consistency, edges and character, biopsies are taken if needed, portahepatis and gastro-hepatic ligaments are inspected and palpated to identify any variations in anatomy, in particular, accessory or replaced hepatic artery branches. In order to flush the preservative solution through liver and kidneys, infra-renal aorta is isolated, looped and cannulated. Similarly, the inferior mesenteric vein (IMV) is cannulated for perfusion. The supra-celiac aorta is clamped to restrict circulation of the solution through the abdominal viscera. Blood from these organs is vented out through the inferior vena cava (IVC). The gallbladder is incised and flushed with saline to prevent cholestasis. The liver is harvested by dividing its attachments. Long lengths of portal structures such as the

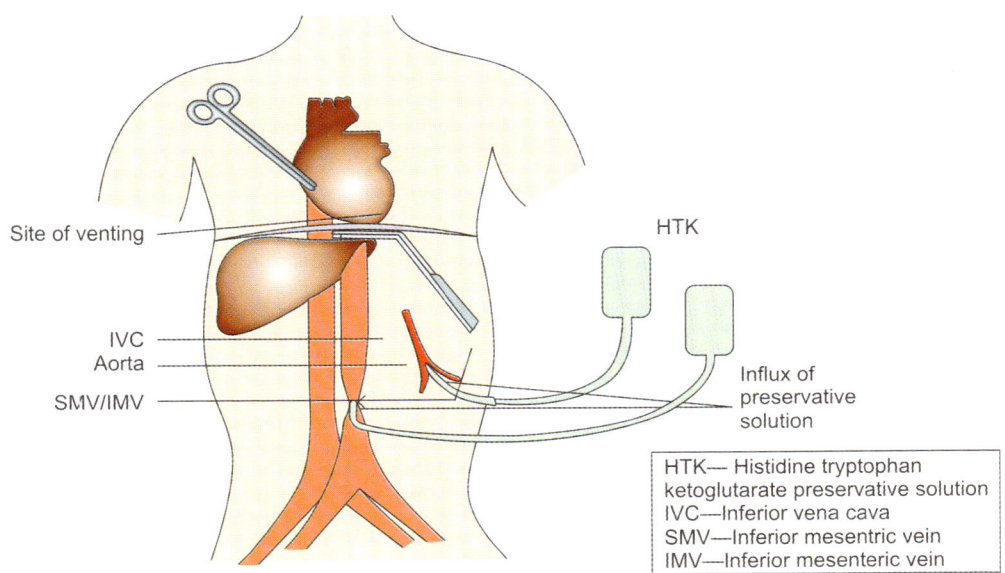

Fig. 16.2: Deceased donor organ recovery

bile duct, hepatic artery and portal vein are preserved with the liver graft and the IVC and aorta are transected above the renal vessels inferiorly and at the level of the diaphragm superiorly. The liver is packed, stored and transported in sterile ice slush for surface cooling. Recovery from a DCD donor is similar, except the need for a rapid aortic cannulation and establishing perfusion quickly with most of the dissection being done in cold phase.

After recovery of the liver, it is re-inspected for gross appearance, uniformity of perfusion, procurement injuries and vascular anatomy. IVC and portal structures are dissected clean from the surrounding tissue. Superior mesenteric artery and left gastric artery (LGA) are examined for accessory hepatic vessels. In case accessory hepatic artery is present a reconstruction is done such that the whole graft is supplied by a common feeder artery. Infrahepatic IVC stump is closed.

Living Donor Hepatectomy

While left lateral segment donation is generally required for pediatric LDLT and right lobe for adult-to-adult living donor liver transplantation (AALDLT, Fig. 16.3), the left lobe may be used for an adolescent or small adult. The liver is mobilized by dividing the round, falciform and ipsilateral triangular ligaments. For right lobe donation, hepatic veins draining the caudate lobe between the right lobe and IVC are divided. Right hepatic vein (RHV) and any large hepatic veins

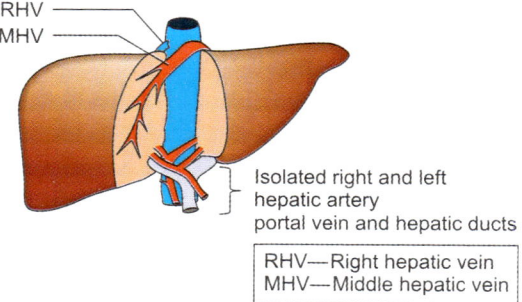

RHV — Right hepatic vein
MHV — Middle hepatic vein

Fig. 16.3: Living donor hepatectomy

draining the right lobe (>5 mm) are preserved. Cholecystectomy and a cholangiogram are done. The common hepatic artery (HA), bile duct and portal vein (PV) are identified and right HA, PV are isolated and temporarily occluded to mark the interlobar ischaemic plane. Liver parenchyma is transected along the ischaemic line using CUSA (Cavitronic ultrasonic suction aspirator). The right hepatic duct, hepatic artery, portal vein and RHV are sequentially divided and the liver is removed and perfused with the preservative solution. Right lobe grafts may be retrieved with or without the middle hepatic vein (MHV). When retrieved without the MHV, major segment 5 and 8 branches may be reconstructed using a PTFE graft or cryopreserved veins.

Laparoscopic or robotic donor hepatectomy is an evolving field and has the benefits of less pain, better cosmetic scar, less wound complications, early recovery and discharge from the hospital. However, it is technically complex and can only be justified in very selected cases with favourable vascular anatomy by a team with a large experience in open and laparoscopic liver surgery.

Recipient Operation

The recipient operation can be broadly divided into the initial phase of recipient native hepatectomy leading to anhepatic phase and implantation of the liver graft resulting in the neohepatic phase.

Recipient Native Hepatectomy

Recipient native hepatectomy may be performed using the classic or piggyback technique. While the classic technique involves resection of native liver together with the retrohepatic IVC attached, the piggyback technique consists of dissection of the caudate and right lobe off the retrohepatic IVC to preserve it in the recipient. Therefore, while the conventional technique allows quicker hepatectomy, piggyback technique maintains haemodynamic stability and preserves renal venous outflow and is more commonly used.

Piggyback technique for recipient native hepatectomy: After adequate exposure, ligamentous attachments of the liver are divided. Hepatic artery, portal vein and bile duct are isolated and divided, preserving long stumps. The liver is dissected off the IVC by dividing the caudate veins. RHV, MHV and left hepatic vein (LHV) are clamped and divided leaving long stumps. Thus, the native liver is explanted without clamping the IVC.

Classic technique of recipient native hepatectomy: Initial steps are as described above. After division of the hilar structures, the IVC is mobilized off the retroperitoneum and right adrenal vein is divided. Suprahepatic and infrahepatic (suprarenal) IVC are mobilized, looped, clamped and divided and the liver is explanted along with the intrahepatic portion of IVC.

During the anhepatic phase, a temporary end to side portocaval shunt may be done if the anhepatic phase is expected to be long or significant bowel congestion is observed like in acute liver failure. Although uncommon, a venovenous bypass (VVB) may be used to reduce the adverse effects of IVC and PV occlusion, especially in patients with renal or cardiac dysfunction.

Liver Allograft Implantation

Implantation of the new liver consists of vascular anastomosis, reperfusion and biliary reconstruction. The graft could be implanted using the conventional or the piggyback technique, the latter being more commonly used.

Whole graft (deceased donor graft) implantation using piggyback technique: In this technique, the supra-hepatic IVC of the liver graft is anastomosed to the stumps of recipient hepatic veins. Alternatively, side-to-side cavoplasty may be done. End-to-end graft and recipient PV anastomosis is done leaving a "growth factor" to prevent PV anastomotic narrowing. The graft is reperfused with recipient portal blood. Reperfusion may cause hemodynamic instability because of hyperkalemia, tissue factors release and loss of systemic resistance. This is followed by hepatic arterial anastomosis under magnification followed by anastomosis of graft bile duct with recipient CBD. In patients with PSC, biliary atresia or some other situations, a hepaticojejunostomy may be required (Fig 16.4).

Partial graft implantation using piggyback technique: A partial graft may be obtained from a living donor or split from a deceased donor. For right lobe implantation, a wide anastomosis is made between the donor RHV and recipient RHV. Any significant inferior HV (> 5 mm) preserved during graft retrieval is anastomosed end-to-side to a separate cavotomy. Graft MHV or segment 5/8 PTFE conduit is anastomosed to recipient LHV/MHV stump. Graft right portal vein (RPV) is anastomosed to recipient PV followed by

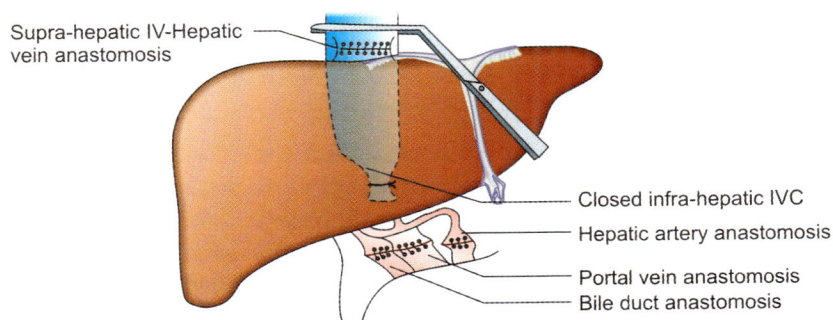

Supra-hepatic IV-Hepatic vein anastomosis

Closed infra-hepatic IVC
Hepatic artery anastomosis
Portal vein anastomosis
Bile duct anastomosis

Fig. 16.4: "Piggyback" technique for whole graft implantation

reperfusion. HA anastomosis is done under magnification followed by bile duct anastomosis (Fig. 16.5).

Alternatives Techniques in Liver Transplantation

Auxiliary Liver Transplantation

Auxiliary partial orthotopic liver transplant involves removal of one-half of native liver enabling placement of an auxiliary partial graft in its place. When done in patients with acute liver failure, where the native liver has the potential for regeneration, it may allow complete withdrawal of immunosuppression. In children, about two-thirds patients can weaned off immunosuppression avoiding their long-term side-effects.

Dual-Lobe Living Donor Liver Transplantation

Living donors are commonly rejected for inadequate estimated graft volume. Dual lobe LDLT allows two donors to donate one lobe each to provide adequate liver mass for one recipient. This is a technically demanding procedure, commonly involves implantation of one right and left lobe or two left lobes.

ABO Incompatible Liver Transplant (ABOi LT)

ABO incompatible liver transplants carry a high-risk of humoral rejection except in infants and small children, who have low antibody titers and an immature complement system. Adults require pre-transplant preparation with rituximab, plasmapheresis and immunosuppression to reduce the ABO antibody titers followed by close monitoring of the same after transplant. The graft undergoes accommodation in few months, after which the risk of humoral rejection is low. Living donor liver transplantation is especially suitable for ABOiLT as it allows time for preparation and antibody reducing strategies to be employed and monitored. It is generally offered to stable patients because of the risk of infection related decompensation in patients with advanced cirrhosis.

Domino Liver Transplantation

In domino liver transplant, the liver removed from the patient undergoing transplant can be used for transplant in another patient. This is possible in certain metabolic diseases like familial amyloid polyneuropathy (FAPN) and maple syrup urine disease (MSUD), because the liver is structurally and functionally normal apart from production of abnormal protein. These livers are preferably used in elderly patients with life-expectancy less than the time needed to develop clinical symptoms from the domino graft.

Paired Donor Exchange/Swap Living Donor Liver Transplantation

Often living donors are medically suitable but blood group incompatible for their recipient. When two such donor-recipient pairs have complimentary blood groups, a paired donor exchange or swap living donor liver transplant is performed. It does not impose any additional risk on individual donors or recipients, although it is logistically more demanding.

POSTOPERATIVE MANAGEMENT, COMPLICATIONS AND OUTCOMES

Post-transplant care involves monitoring of haemodynamic, clinical and laboratory parameters, timely detection and management of complications and balanced immuno-suppression to prevent graft rejection and avoid infection. Signs of improving liver graft function include improving sensorium, lactate

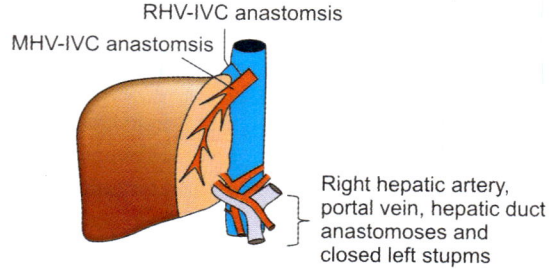

RHV-IVC anastomsis

MHV-IVC anastomsis

Right hepatic artery, portal vein, hepatic duct anastomoses and closed left stupms

Fig. 16.5: Living donor right lobe liver graft implantation

levels, INR/bilirubin and decreasing trend of liver injury enzymes, SGOT and SGPT. Patients receive prophylactic antibiotics, antifungal and antiviral medications, *Pneumocystis jeroveci* (carinii) prophylaxis with sulphamethoxazole/trimethoprim, CMV prophylaxis for high-risk individuals, ulcer prophylaxis with a proton pump inhibitor, low-dose aspirin for anti-coagulation, vitamin and mineral supplements and drugs for pre-existing comorbidities. In addition to graft function, immunosuppressive drug levels are monitored. Patients are advised to follow safe hygienic practices and to avoid contact with sick individuals.

Immunosuppression. Its regimen and protocols are not uniform across the world and continue to evolve with availability of newer drugs. The goal is to provide effective immunosuppression against allograft rejection while preserving immunologic control of infection and neoplasms and minimizing their long-term toxicity. Immunosuppression regimen consists of an induction phase followed by life-long maintenance phase.Induction is generally done with a bolus dose of steroids or rarely using one of the interleukin-2 receptor (IL-2R) or T-cell depleting antibodies followed by maintenance with combination of two or more drugs including calcineurin inhibitors (CNIs), antiproliferative agents, mammalian target of rapamycin (mTOR) inhibitors and steroids (Table 16.6). The selection of agents is based on an individual's medical history as well as on institutional experience and preference. In patients with renal dysfunction, induction with an IL-2R antibody allows CNI sparing in early postoperative period. Patients with autoimmune hepatitis (AIH) need higher drug levels and life-long low-dose steroids to prevent rejection and disease recurrence. Patients with HCC may benefit from sirolimus-based regimens to reduce risk of recurrence. Pediatric patients benefit from IL-2R antibody induction and need rapid tapering of steroids to avoid adverse influence on growth.

While early (first 3 months) complications are generally due to technical aspects of the operation (i.e. vascular and biliary complications), graft quality and infections (Table 16.7), those in intermediate period (3–12 months) are due to rejection and opportunistic infections and late ones (after 12 months) because of long-term drug toxicity, biliary stricture, recurrent disease, malignancy [skin cancers, post-transplant lymphoproliferative disease (PTLD), etc.], cardiorespiratory, cerebrovascular and chronic rejection.

Primary nonfunction (PNF). It is uncommon (DDLT: 4.6–9%, LDLT: 0.3%), but potentially life-threatening complication. It is characterized by encephalopathy, minimal bile production, hyperbilirubinaemia, coagulopathy, rapidly rising AST/ALT and increasing lactate. Donor risk factors such as advanced age, moderate to severe steatosis, prolonged cold ischaemia time, high serum sodium and DCD have been implicated as causative factors. Patients with PNF are given priority on the waiting list for an emergency re-transplant.

Small for size syndrome (SFSS). It is a syndrome of hyperbilirubenaemia, ascites and coagulopathy seen in patients who receive small grafts (GRWR <0.8). However, factors such as poor graft quality (moderate to severe steatosis, fibrosis) or portal hyperperfusio nare also known to cause SFSS. Portal hyperperfusion may be prevented by using vasoactive drugs (somatostatin or vasopressin analogs), splenectomy, splenic artery ligation, hemiportocaval shunt.

Hepatic artery thrombosis (HAT). It is seen in children (6–8%) and in LDLT more than adults (4%) and DDLT. It may present with dramatic increase in liver function tests (LFTs), bile leak or more commonly diagnosed on protocol Doppler ultrasonography (DUS). A resistive index (RI) of less than 0.5, systolic acceleration time (SAT) greater than 150 ms or parvustardus waveform on DUS are indicative of HAT. On suspicion, a tri-phasic CT scan is done for confirmation followed by either an emergency

	Table 16.6: Immunosuppressive drugs			
Group	Name (preparations)	Mechanism of action	Side effects	Doses/target levels
Calcineurin inhibitors (CNI)	Cyclosporine (cyclosporin A, microemulsified Neoral)	Suppresses activation of T lymphocytes by blocking production of interleukin-2 (IL-2) and other lymphokines via cyclophilin	• Hypertension • Renal dysfunction • Hirsutism • Hyperkalaemia • Gum hyperplasia	10–15 mg/kg/day in two doses (target 250–350 ng/mL)
	Tacrolimus (sustained-release Advagraf)	Suppresses activation of T-lymphocytes by blocking production of IL-2 and other lympho-kines by binding to T-cell FK binding protein (FKBP 12)	• Tremor • Diabetes mellitus • Hyperkalaemia • Hypertension • Headache • Renal dysfunction	0.15–0.3 mg/kg/day (target 8–10 ng/mL)
Corticosteroids	Methylprednisolone/ Wysolone	• Causes emigration of T-cells from intravascular to lymphoid tissues • Blocks activation of T-cells and anti-gen presenting cells (APCs) by inactivating nuclear factor • Inhibits cytokine transcription by APC	• Diabetes • Cardiovascular problems • Myopathy • Peptic ulcer • Impaired wound healing • Ocular problems (cataract/glaucoma)	250–1,000 mg at the time of transplant as induction dose and then 1 mg/kg/day as maintenance and tapering of dose thereafter
Nucleoside inhibitor	Azathioprine Mycophenolate-mofetil (MMF) MMF potassium-Cellcept MMF Sodium-Myfortic	Inhibits purine synthesis and differentiation and proliferation of T- and B-lymphocytes	• Cytopenia (bone marrow suppression) • Gastrointestinal disturbance (less with Myfortic)	3–5 mg/kg orally or IV once a day 150–600 mg/m²/dose
mTOR inhibitors	Sirolimus	• Binds to FKBP12 which inhibits activation of mammalian target of rapamycin (mTOR) regula-tory kinase	• Early hepatic artery thrombosis (HAT) • Dyslipidemia • Proteinuria • Cytopenia	6 mg followed by a maintenance dose of 2 mg given once daily (target 5–12 ng/mL)
	Everolimus	• Inhibits T lymphocyte activation and proliferation by IL-2, IL-4 and IL-5		1.5–2 mg in divided doses target 3–8 ng/mL

(Contd.)

Table 16.6: Immunosuppressive drugs (Contd.)

Group	Name (preparations)	Mechanism of action	Side-effects	Doses/target levels
T and B-cell receptor antibodies	Basiliximab (chimeric)	• IL-2 receptor antagonist by binding with high affinity to alpha chain of IL-2 receptors complex and inhibit IL-2 binding	• Acne • Gastrointestinal disturbance • Tremor	20 mg on the day of surgery and 20 mg after 4 days
	Daclizumab (humanized)	• Competitive antagonism of IL-2-induced T-cell proliferation	• Back pain • Gastrointestinal disturbance • Impaired wound healing • Pedal oedema	1 mg/kg every 14 days (total five doses)
	Thymoglobulin (ATG)	Antibodies against multiple thymocyte surface antigens. Depletes circulating T-lymphocytes, modulates their activation, homing and cytotoxicity	• Cytokine release syndrome • First-dose effect (ranges from flu-like symptoms to pulmonary oedema	1.5–5 mg/kg as a single infusion usually over 4–6 hours for 3–5 days
	OKT3 (Muromonab-CD3)	Directed against CD3 complex, inacti-vates and depletes T-lymphocytes		5 mg intravenously daily for 10–14 days
	Alemtuzumab	Directed against CD52, depletes lymphocytes, natural killer cells and monocytes	Flu-like symptoms	30 mg perioperati-vely

Table 16.7: Post-transplant complications

Early (< 3 months)	Intermediate (3-12 months)	Late (> 12 months)
• Bleeding • Vascular complications • Primary graft nonfunction • Infections/bacterial sepsis • Small for size syndrome • Biliary leak • Rejection • Perforated viscus • Surgical site infections • CMV infection	• Biliary strictures • Hepatic vein stenosis • Rejection • EBV infection, PTLD • Hypertension • Poor growth	• PTLD • Late biliary strictures • Renal dysfunction • Hypertension • Noncompliance with medications • NODM • Recurrence (HCV, HBV, HCC) • Unusual infections • Cancer • Growth failure • Osteopenia • Hernia (incisional and others)

Abbreviations: CMV, cytomegalovirus; EBV, Epstein-Barr virus; PTLD, post-transplant lymphoproliferative disease; NODM, new-onset diabetes mellitus; HBV, hepatitis B virus; HCV, hepatitis C virus; HCC, hepatocellular carcinoma.

thrombolysis or surgical revision of the arterial anastomosis or re-transplantation. Late HAT (>3 weeks) may present with biliary complications or a patient with chronic HAT may form collaterals.

Hepatic artery stenosis. (>50% reduction in caliber on angiography) may be encountered in about 5% patients.They may be clinically silent or present with multiple biliary strictures and intermittent bacteremia and may need radiological stenting.

Portal vein thrombosis (PVT). It is more commonly seen in children (3–7%). PVT can present as graft dysfunction and massive ascites, and is diagnosed on DUS or CT angiography. Early PVT is best treated by immediate surgical thrombectomy and revision while late PVT or portal vein stenosis is better treated with percutaneous transhepatic stenting.

Hepatic venous outflow obstruction (HVOO). It may manifest as graft dysfunction, massive ascites, bleeding or even graft rupture. It may be amenable to transjugular angioplasty, pressure gradient measurement and stenting.

Bile leak. (12–34%) may be early (<4 weeks) or late. Early bile leak is commonly anastomotic or from the cut surface in partial grafts. While most of them may stop spontaneously, for large leaks endoscopic sphincterotomy and biliary stenting or conversion to hepaticojejunostomy may be required.

Biliary strictures. These (4–16%) are more common in LDLT, can be anastomotic or non-anastomotic/diffuse. Anastomotic strictures are usually early and managed with endoscopic balloon dilatation and stenting or percutaneous transhepatic dilatation and stenting (in patients with Roux-en-Y anastomosis) with periodic stent exchanges until stricture is remodeled. Failed attempts at interventional techniques may need surgical revision or conversion to Roux- en-Y biliary anastomosis. Diffuse

intrahepatic strictures may be due to severe preservation injury, ischaemic insult or hepatic arterial insufficiency and may warrant a retransplant.

Acute cellular allograft rejection (ACR). It is commonly caused by T-cells that get activated by direct or indirect pathways, various immunosuppressive drugs used after transplant, block one of these pathways (Fig. 16.6). Liver is resilient to antibody mediated rejection compared to other organs. ACR may be encountered in as many as 20–40% patients within the first 3–6 months and may be as high as 50–70% in children. It may present with fever, jaundice, abdominal pain or raised AST/ALT, although these are non-specific and histological confirmation is needed. Lymphocytic infiltration in portal triads, venous endothelial inflammation and bile duct damage are seen on histology, graded using rejection activity index (RAI) and used to guide therapy. With current immunosuppression protocols, graft loss secondary to rejection is uncommon.

Chronic rejection. It is uncommon (2–5%) and may occur following multiple episodes of recurrent acute rejection or de novo mostly due to poor compliance. It is characterized by slowly progressive clinical and biochemical signs of cholestasis, bile duct paucity (ductopenia) on histopathology and may lead to graft loss and require retransplantation.

Infections. They are common after transplant and may be divided into early (<1 month), intermediate (1–6 months) and late (>6 months) (Table 16.8), even though patients are vaccinated against common infections and receive prophylactic antibiotics, antifungals and antiviral medications. Infectious complications (29–56%) are the most common causes of morbidity and mortality after transplant; therefore, close surveillance, early evaluation and timely therapy should be instituted, especially because immunosuppression may mask common signs of infection and predispose to atypical infections. Serious bacterial

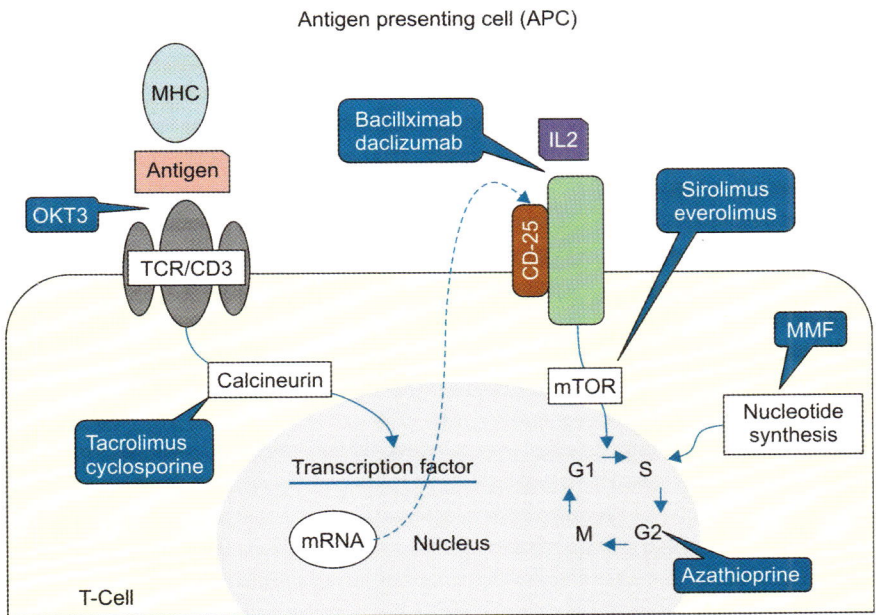

Fig. 16.6: Mechanism of action of various immunosuppressive drugs

Table 16.8: Timeline of infections in the post-transplant period		
Early (<1 month)	*Intermediate (1–6 months)*	*Late (>6 months)*
Pneumonia	Legionella	VZV
Urinary tract infections	TB	CMV retinitis
IV Catheter related infections	Listeria	Legionella
Wound infections	Nocardia	Listeria
Candida, aspergillus	CMV, HHV6, EBV, adenovirus	Toxoplasmosis
VRE	Toxoplasmosis	Histoplasma
C.Difficile	Candida	Coccidioidomycosis
HSV	Aspergillus	JC/BK virus
	Histoplasma	Pneumocystis
	Cryptococcus	Cryptococcus
	Pneumocystis	
	Coccidioidomycosis	
	Hepatitis B and C	

Abbreviations: HSV Herpes simplex virus, CMV—Cytomegalovirus, HHV—Human herpes virus, EBV—Ebstein-Barr virus, VZV—Varicella zoster virus.

infections may occur in about one-third of patients requiring temporary reduction or cessation of immunosuppression with appropriate antimicrobial therapy. Intermediate infections are often opportunistic in nature such as Cytomegalovirus (CMV), Herpes simplex viral (HSV), *Pneumocystis jeroveci* (carinii) pneumonia or atypical infections such as *Aspergillus*, Nocardia, Listeria, Cryptococcus, *Mycobacterium tuberculosis*, respiratory syncytial virus (RSV), human herpes virus 6 (HHV-6), influenza, adenovirus and Epstein-Barr virus (EBV). Late infections are commonly community acquired such as pneumonia and urinary infection with organisms like Legionella, Listeria, Cryptococcus, Histoplasma, Coccidioides and Blastomyces.

Metabolic complications. Complications such as hypercholesterolemia, obesity, new onset post-transplant diabetes mellitus (NODM, PTDM), hypertension, hyperuricemia, osteoporosis is seen in 15–45% of patients over years after transplant. Immunosuppressive medicines, especially steroids and CNIs are contributory factors and may improve with change to another mTOR inhibitors or steroid withdrawal.

Renal dysfunction. It occurs in 4–9% of the transplant recipients mainly related to the use of calcineurin inhibitors, presence of pre-transplant renal dysfunction and other renal diseases.

Skin and lymphoid malignancies. These malignancies are common with incidence up to 40% and 10% respectively. Post-transplant lymphoproliferative disease (PTLD) has a strong association with EBV infection. It may present with non-specific symptoms such as fever, localized or disseminated lymph nodes enlargement or solid tumors. Treatment involves cessation or reduction of immunosuppression, surgical removal of tumors, ganciclovir, anti-CD20 monoclonal-antibody, rituximab, and systemic chemotherapy.

Disease recurrence. It is now uncommon in HBV and HCV infections, but PSC, PBC or AIH recurrence risk is about 15% at 3 years to 30% at 10 years.

Outcomes

Overall patient and graft survival depends on the type of transplant (DDLT vs. LDLT), type of deceased donor (Ideal, ECD, DCD) and recipient age (pediatric, adult). Typically 1 and 5 year patient survival is 85–90% and 75–80% and graft survival is 75–80% and 70–75%, respectively. Results are comparable between DDLT and LDLT but inferior with DCD grafts.

Patients have a good quality of life, resume work in a few months. Pregnancy is safe after transplant with modification of immunosuppressive regimen. Children have catch-up growth and good academic progress in the long-term.

Legal Issues

The transplantation of human organs (THOA) act was passed in 1994 that outlined the legal framework for transplant activity in India. The law defines the infrastructure, equipment and manpower requirements and the process for a hospital to obtain a license for transplantation by the appropriate authority. It identifies brainstem death and defines the criteria and procedure for certification of the same by the brain death committee. The law defines the process to be followed for living donor transplant and empowers authorization committee to examine and approve each transplant case to prevent organ trading. Strict penalties for any violation of the law have also been defined.

Summary

Liver transplantation is the standard of care for all types of end stage liver disease and acute liver failure. The major limiting factor is organ scarcity. Even with utilization of marginal donors, split liver transplants and LDLT's, there is a huge gap between demand and supply.

17

Splenomegaly

Alaka Deshpande

Spleen is a reticuloendothelial organ, 12 × 7 cm in size, encapsulated lying entirely within the rib cage located in the left hypochondrium. It is attached to stomach by gastrolineal ligament and with the left kidney by lienorenal ligament. It is supplied by a splenic artery and drained by a splenic vein which together with superior mesentric vein forms the portal vein. The development of spleen is from dorsal mesogastrium at about five weeks of gestation. It arises in a series of hillocks which unify in a single tissue mass, i.e. spleen. If the hillocks fail to unify 20% of the people have an accessory spleen. It has a red and a white pulp centred around small branches of the splenic artery. The red pulp is red blood filled sinuses and cords lined by reticuloendothelial (RE) cells. While white pulp is lymphoid follicles arrayed in the red pulp.

Functions of the Spleen

1. Removal of senescent and defective RBCs and maintenance of the quality control of the red cells.
2. Antibody synthesis by white pulp.
3. Removal of antibody coated bacteria and antibody coated blood cells from the circulation.

Clinically, a palpable spleen indicates its enlargement in many disease conditions.

Palpation of the Spleen

The patient is asked to take a deep breath. The abdominal palpation is started from the right iliac fossa towards the left costal margin. The tip of the enlarged spleen touches the palpating fingers during inspiration. The size, the surface, the consistency (soft or firm), presence of tenderness and the splenic notch are noted. Spleen to be clinically palpable has to be enlarged 2.5 to 3 times its normal size. In case of clinically impalpable spleen, the size can be assessed by abdominal ultrasonography.

Clinically the Splenomegaly can be Classified as:

Mild just palpable spleen, up to 5 cm below the left costal margin.

Moderate splenomegaly up to umbilicus.

Massive beyond umbilicus, reaching up to the right iliac fossa.

Causes of Mild Splenomegaly

Infections

Bacterial—Typhoid, paratyphoid, septicaemia, subacute bacterial endocarditis, meningococcemia, tuberculosis.

Viral infections—Acute viral hepatitis, cytomegalovirus, HIV, infectious mononucleosis.

Parasitic—Acute malaria, acute *kala azar*, trypanosomiasis, amoebic hepatitis.

Fungal—Histoplasmosis

Hematological Conditions

Iron deficiency anaemia, megaloblastic anaemia, aplastic anaemia, acute idiopathic thrombocytopenia, acute leukaemia, immune neutropenia.

Collagen Vascular Diseases

SLE, PAN, Rheumatoid arthritis.

Other Conditions

Sarcoidosis, amyloidosis.

Moderate Splenomegaly up to Umbilicus

- Portal hypertension
- Inherited hemolytic anaemia
  - Hereditary spherocytosis
  - Sickle cell disease
- Autoimmune hemolytic anaemia
- Chronic lymphatic leukaemia (B-Cell)
- Hodgkin's lymphoma
- Polycythemia vera

Massive Splenomegaly Beyond Umbilicus

- Chronic myeloid leukaemia
- Thalassemia major
- Myelosclerosis with myeloid metaplasia
- Storage disorders
  - Gaucher's disease
  - Niemann-Pick disease
- Splenic cyst
- Splenic tumours

Salient Clinical Features

Mild Splenomegaly

The causes of mild splenomegaly enlisted above have a characteristic clinical profile of the primay ailment. A presence of mild splenomegaly is a part and parcel of the clinical profile of the disease condition and thus helps in diagnosis. These conditions have just palpable, soft splenomegaly. It recedes with successful treatment of the condition.

Moderate Splenomegaly

The spleen is enlarged up to umbilicus. Patient at the time of presentation may have complaints only due to splenomegaly per se such as a lump in the left side of the abdomen, fullness of stomach after small meals, occasionally dragging pain in the left hypochondrium. In addition patient may have features of the disease which has caused the spleen to enlarge.

Massive Splenomegaly

Spleen is enlarged beyond umbilicus reaching almost right iliac fossa. The mere size of the spleen gives an appearance of distension of the abdomen. It causes dragging pain. It is also vulnerable to traumatic rupture. In addition signs and symptoms of underlying condition are present.

One has to determine the aetiology of this splenomegaly. The salient clinical features of each condition are briefly described below for differential diagnosis.

Moderate Splenomegaly

Portal Hypertension (PHT)

Patient may present with or give history of haematemesis from bleeding varices. Other signs of portosystemic collaterals may be present.

The most common aetiology of portal hypertension is cirrhosis of the liver which is commonly due to chronic alcoholism or HBV/HCV infection.

1. History of chronic alcoholism should be inquired.
2. Stigmata of cirrhosis may be present, e.g. jaundice, clubbing, spider naevi, gynecomastia, palmer erythema, ascites or signs of hepatic encephalopathy.
3. Patient should be examined for evidence related to other causes of portal hypertension.

Relevant investigations include:

1. Liver function tests: Reversal of Alb/Glob ratio in cirrhosis

   Increased prothrombin time
2. Upper GI scopy: for evidence of oesophageal and fundal varices

3. Abdominal sonography: One can document
   - splenomegaly
   - the diameter of the portal vein,
   - collateral channels,
   - echotexture of the liver suggesting cirrhosis,
   - presence of ascites,
   - any evidence of causes of portal hypertension other than cirrhosis, e.g. portal hemangioma, portal vein thrombosis, etc.

Treat the cause and treat the complications of PHT.

Inherited Haemolytic Anaemia

Moderate splenomegaly is seen in haemolytic anaemia as the spleen removes the defective RBCs.

The defect may be in the RBC membrane or haemoglobin.

Three major causes of congenital haemolytic anemia are:
   - Hereditary spherocytosis (membrane cyto-skeleton defect)
   - Sickle cell disease (haemoglobinpathy, autosplenectomy is common)
   - Thalassemia major (haemoglobinopathy, massive splenomegaly)

Hereditary Spherocytosis

Young patient may present with history of repeated attacks of mild jaundice, similar history in the siblings, mild anaemia and gallstones. Splenomegaly is moderate.

Unconjugated bilirubin is more than conjugated bilirubin in the serum.

Peripheral smear of the blood shows spherical RBCs.

The classical features is increased MCHC.

The diagnosis is confirmed by osmotic fragility test. The RBC with membrane defect are lysed at a higher osmolality.

The treatment is splenectomy.

Sickle cell disease. It is due to haemoglobino-pathy. The aminoacid at position 6 in globin is normally glutamic acid which is substituted by valine. This abnormal haemoglobin is HbS. In circumstances of dehydration, deoxygenation and acidosis, the HbS polymerizes and precipitates in the RBCs taking a form of sickle. The sickled cells lose the pliability needed to traverse the smaller capillaries. They are abnormally adherent to the endothelium of small venules causing veno occlusion and pre-mature RBC destruction. The rigid adherent cells clog small capillaries and venules resulting into ischaemia and infarction of tissue.

Spleen is the organ lysing RBCs hence there is a splenomegly but repeated micro-infracts in spleen having microvascular bed cause autolysis in first 18–36 months of life (auto-splenectomy).

The homozygous inheritance presents as a sickle cell disease while heterozygous show sickle cell trait with mild anaemia and absence of vaso-occulusive manifestations.

Investigation

- Anaemia,
- peripheral smear showing sickled RBCs
- increased reticulocyte count.
- Na-metabisulphite test precipitating sickling phenomenon.
- Hb electrophoresis for haemoglobin S.
- Genotyping of family members.

Mainstay of Management

- Hydration
- Hydroxyurea 10–30 mg/kg/day
- Bone marrow transplantation

Autoimmune Haemolytic Anaemia

It is an acquired disorder caused by autoantibody directed against a red cell antigen. The autoantibody binds to the red cell. Once the red cell is coated with autoantibody it will be destroyed. In majority of the cases Fc portion of the antibody is recongnized by Fc receptor of the macrophages and this triggers erythrophagocytosis. The spleen has abundant macrophages, so are liver and bone marrow.

However, due to unique anatomy of the spleen, antibody coated red cells are trapped more efficiently in the spleen and destroyed. It is also known extravascular haemolysis.

It is usually seen in the middle age. The onset is often abrupt. The haemoglobin level drops acutely, jaundice may appear due to massive red cell destruction. Spleen is enlarged. Acute onset anaemia without apparent cause, jaundice and splenomegaly in a middle aged person raises high suspicion of autoimmune haemolytic anaemia.

The diagnosis is established by Coomb's test. The cause remains obscure. A full screen of autoimmune disease can be carried out.

Severe acute autoimmune haemolytic anaemia is a medical emergency. Blood transfusion is an immediate treatment. Due to presence of antibodies, cross matching poses problems. Being an autoimmune disorder, prednisolone 1 mg/kg/day may produce prompt remission. Spleen being the major site of RBC destruction splenectomy was advocated in the past though it does not cure the condition. The availability of rituximab, is a good alternative to splenectomy. The immunosuppressants like azathioprine, cyclosporine, IVIG are third line drugs.

Stem cell transplantation has been used successfully.

B-Cell Chronic Lymphatic Leukaemia

Table shows the staging of typical B-cell CLL (Table 17.1).

Rai stage 0 and Binet stage A can be followed without specific therapy.

Intermmediate stage: Disease manifested with lymphadenopathy and/or hepatospleno-megaly require treatment in first few years of follow-up.

Advanced stage: Rai stage III or Binet stage C requires therapy. Chlorambucil administered orally or fludarabine give IV are used for treatment.

Combination of rituximab 375–500 mg/m^2 day 1 + fludarabine(25 mg/m^2 days 2–4 of cycle 1 and day 1–3 of subsequent cycles) and(cyclophosphamide 250 mg/m^2 with fludarabine) achieves remission in more than 69% of cases.

Hodgkin's Lymphoma

Hodgkin's disease can present with non-tender lymphadenopathy in neck, supracla-vicular area, axilla, mediastinum or abdomen in older patients.

Patient may present with pyrexia of unknown origin. A few patients may present with relapsing type of Pel-Ebstein's type of fever. Ann Arbor staging system is used. The diagnosis is established by lymph node FNAC/biopsy.

Table 17.1: Staging of B-cell CLL		
Stage	*Clinical profile*	*Mean survival in years*
Rai System		
O Low-risk	Lymphocytosis only in blood and bone marrow	10
I Intermediate-risk	Lymphocytosis + lymphadenopathy	7 years
II Intermediate-risk	Lymphocytosis + lymphadenopathy+splenomegaly/ hepatomegaly	
III High-risk	Lymphocytosis + anaemia	1.5 years
IV High-risk	Lymphocytosis +Thrombocytopaenia	
Binet system		
A	LN enlargement at <3 sites	10 years
B	Lymphadenopathy at >3 sites	7 years
C	B +Hb<10 g/dll + platelets <100,000/μl	1.5 years

Mainstay of the treatment is radiotherapy and chemotherapy. Localized Hodgkin's disease is cured in >90% cases by extended field radiotherapy alternatively, a brief course of chemotherapy followed by radiotherapy is advised. Popular chemotherapy includes:

ABVD: Doxorubicin, bleomycin, vinblastine and dacarbazine

MOPP: Mechlorethamine

Vincristine, procarbazine

And prednisolone

Polycythemia Vera. It is a myeloproliferative disorder without any stimulus. It is a clonal disorder involving pleuripotent progenitor cells of haemopoietic system.

A patient may present with elevated haemoglobin and haematocrit (erythrocytosis), leucocytosis and thrombocytosis or may present with proliferation of one line only.

He can present with splenomegaly. Erythrocytosis with raised Hb cause hyperviscosity resulting into neurological manifestations like throbbing headache, visual disturbances, vertigo, TIAs, etc. Vessels of other systems also are affected. Erythromelagia, hepatic vein thrombosis, digital ischaemia are due to thrombocytosis. Hyperuricemia and secondary gout due to a large turnover of hemopoietic cells is seen.

It is an indolent disorder. Thrombosis due to erythrocytosis is a common complication. The Hb level should be maintained < 14 gm/dl and haematocrit (Hct) <45% by repeated phlebotomies.

Use of radioactive phosphorus P32, or other alkylating agents are leukemogenic and should be used only in consultation with haematologist.

Massive Splenomegaly

Chronic Myeloid Leukaemia (CML)

Myloid Leukaemias are a hetetrogenous group of diseases characterized by malignant infiltration of blood, bone marrow and other tissues by malignant cells of hemopoietic system.

CML is due to clonal expansion of hemopoietic stem cells possessing a reciprocal translocation between chromosome 9 and 22.

Initially, the cells of myeloid series show certain degree of maturation so the peripheral blood has immature cells like myelocytes and metamyelocytes, with elevated total WBC count. The WBC count varies from 100,000 to 500,000/mm^3. The bone marrow cellularity is increased with an increase in myeloid/erythroid ratio. The blast cell percentage in the beginning is almost normal.

If untreated, the disease shows transition from the chronic phase to an accelerated phase of blast crisis. Clinically, the onset of the chronic phase is commonly in the middle age and is insiduous. Patient may present with fatigue, malaise. He may present with symptoms related to splenomegaly such as early satiety, mass in the left hypochondrium or dragging pain in the left hypochondrium. Platelet dysfunction may present with occasional bleeding gums. Severe leucocytosis may result into vaso-occlusive disease leading to venous thrombosis, cerebrovascular accidents, priapism, visual disturbances, etc. Clinical examination shows massive splenomegaly, mild anaemia.

At the time of diagnosis of a chronic phase, the WBC count is elevated (>100,000 to 500,000/mm^3) with increase in both immature as well as mature cells.

Bone marrow cellularity is increased with almost normal percentage of blast cells.

Disease acceleration from chronic to acute stage is marked by increased anaemia with blast cells up to 20% in blood and the marrow. When the blast cells are > 20% it is defined as blast crisis.

Cytogenetic study shows Philadelphia chromosome in 90–95% of cases. (Shortened chromosome 22 (22q-) which arises from reciprocal t(9;22).

The cytogenetic hallmark of CML is t(9;22)(q34;q11.2).

Treatment

In a newly diagnosed case, imatinib 400 mg/day has shown complete hematologic remission rate to be 95%.

Thalassemia

Thalassemia syndromes are inherited disorders resulting into defective bio-synthesis of globin chains of haemoglobin. The genetic mutation can affect any step of gene expression like transcription, translation or post-translational metabolism of polypeptide chains.

The normal adult haemoglobin has 2α and 2β chains of globin moiety. The variants are:

Hb A1	$\alpha_2 \beta_2$
Hb A2	$\alpha_2 \delta_2$
Hb F	$\alpha_2 \gamma_2$
Hb E	$\alpha_2 \beta_2$ 26Glu-Lys
Hb Lepore	$\alpha_2 (\delta\beta)_2$
Hb S	$\alpha_2 \beta_2^{6\ valin}$

The synthesis of the unaffected chain proceeds at a normal rate while there is accumulation of subunits of defective chain. The clinical phenotype is determined by unbalanced chain accumulation.

The homozygous state for the α-thalassemia causes total absence of α-globin synthesis. Physiogiclly useful haemoglobin is not produced beyond embryonic stage resulting into a hydrops foetalis.

β-Thalassemia. The α-chain synthesis is normal. Defective β-chains are substituted by γ-chains therefore even after birth there is more of haemoglobin F-foetal $\alpha2\gamma2$-which is not compatible in postnatal life. Therefore, patient remains anaemic, suffers from growth failure and massive splenomegaly. Unbalanced accumulation of α- and β-chains cause accumulation of highly insoluble α-chains. They form toxic inclusion bodies which affect erythroblasts in the marrow. The RBCs show inclusion bodies. Profound anaemia causes masses of extra-medullary erythropoiesis in the liver and spleen. Clinical features are determined by signs of growth failure, inanition, thlassemic facies with frontal bossing, maxillary marrow hyperplasia, susceptibility to infections, etc. Patient survives with chronic hypertransfusion with iron chelation.

Myelosclerosis with myeloid metaplasia. It is a clonal disorder of multipotent hemopoietic progenitor cells of unknown etiology. It is characterized by myelofibrosis with extra-medullary hematopoiesis and massive splenomegaly.

Gaucher's disease. It is the autosomal recessive storage disorder common in Ashenazi Jews. It usually presents in the late childhood with massive hepato-splenomegaly, respiratory, neurological and bone disease. Large multinucleated Gaucher's cells are identified in the marrow.

Niemann-Pick disease. It also is a storage disorder associated with sphingomyelin storage. It presents with hepatosplenomegaly, infantile neuro-degeneration and failure to thrive.

Splenic cysts and tumours are rarity.

18

General Consideration in Pancreatitis Diseases

Alaka Deshpande, SG Chauhan

The pancreas is an important organ in the abdomen having exocrine as well as endocrine functions. It is located in the retroperitoneum situated transversely across the posterior wall of the abdomen, at the back of the epigastric and left hypochondriac regions. It extends from the second part of the duodenum to the spleen. Its length varies from 12.5 to 15 cm and its weight varies from 60 to 100 gm. Its right extremity, is broader and encircled by the duodenum called the head, and is connected to the main portion of the organ, i.e. body by a light constriction, the neck; while its left extremity gradually tapers to form the tail. It is a compound racemose gland, analogous in its structures to the salivary glands, though softer and less compactly arranged than those organs. The pancreatic acinar cells are grouped into lobules, forming the ductal system which eventually joins the main pancreatic duct.

The pancreatic duct (ductus pancreaticus [Wirsungi]; duct of Wirsung) extends transversely from the left to the right through the substance of the pancreas. It commences by the junction of the small ducts of the lobules situated in the tail of the pancreas, and, running from left to right through the body, it receives the ducts of the various lobules composing the gland. Considerably augmented in size, it reaches the neck, and turning downward, backward, and to the right, it comes into relation with the common bile duct, which lies to its right side. It leaves the head of the gland, passes very obliquely through the mucous and muscular coats of the duodenum, and ends by an orifice common to it and the common bile duct upon the summit of the duodenal papilla, situated at the medial side of the descending portion of the duodenum. It is 7.5 to 10 cm below the pylorus. The pancreatic duct, near the duodenum, is about the size of an ordinary quill. Sometimes the pancreatic duct and the common bile duct open separately into the duodenum. Frequently there is an additional duct, which is given off from the pancreatic duct in the neck of the pancreas and opens into the duodenum about 2.5 cm above the duodenal papilla. It receives the ducts from the lower part of the head, and is known as the accessory pancreatic duct (duct of Santorini). This duct then branches extensively and an acinus lined by secreting cells, cells that carryout the exocrine functions of the pancreas. They are columnar in shape and present two zones: an outer one, clear and finely striated next to the basement membrane, and an inner granular one next to the lumen.

The connective tissue between the alveoli presents collections of cells in certain parts, which are termed interalveolar cell islets (islets of Langerhans). The cells of these islets stain lightly with hematoxylin or carmine, and are more or less polyhedral in shape, forming a network in which ramify many capillaries. There are two main types of cells in the islets, distinguished as A-cells and B-cells according to the special staining reactions of the granules they contain. The islet cells secrete hormones like insulin, glucagon and other hormones.

The arterial supply of the pancreas is derived from the splenic and pancreatic oduodenal branches of the hepatic and superior mesenteric arteries. Pancreas is drained into the splenic and superior mesenteric veins.

FUNCTIONS

The pancreas contains exocrine glands that produce enzymes important to digestion. They include:

Trypsin and chymotrypsin_to digest proteins

Amylase_digestion of carbohydrates

Lipase to breakdown fats.

The pancreatic juices and bile that are released into the duodenum, help the body to digest fats, carbohydrates, and proteins.

Endocrine Function

Approximately three million cell clusters called pancreatic islets are present in the pancreas. The islets function independently from the digestive role played by the majority of pancreatic cells.

Within these islets are four types of cells which are responsible for secretion of hormones. Each type of cell secretes a different type of hormone:

α-alpha cells secrete glucagon (increases blood glucose level)

β-beta cells secrete insulin (decreases blood glucose level)

δ-delta cells secrete somatostatins (regulates/stops α and β-cells), and

PP cells, or γ (gamma) cells, secrete pancreatic polypeptide. These act to control blood glucose through secreting glucagon to increase the levels of glucose, and insulin to decrease it.

Activity of the cells in the islets is under the control of autonomic nervous system.

19

Acute Pancreatitis

Viral Patrawala

Acute pancreatitis is an inflammatory condition of the pancreas clinically characterized by abdominal pain and elevated levels of pancreatic enzymes in the blood.

Acute pancreatitis is defined as inflammation of pancreas which was functionally and structurally normal prior to the attack.

Aetiology

- Gallstone disease and biliary sludge
- Alcohol, methanol, scorpion venom, organophosphate poisoning
- Hyperlipidemia
- Hypercalcaemia
- Drugs—Didanosine, pentamidine, metronidazole, tetracycline, furosemide, thiazides, azathioprines, valproic acid, sulindac, 5-ASA, L-asparaginase, sulphasalazine, salicylates, calcium, oestrogen
- Infections:
    - Viruses—Mumps, Coxsackie, hepatitis B, CMV, Varicella-zoster, HSV, HIV
    - Bacteria—Mycoplasma, Legionella, Leptospira, Salmonella
    - Fungi—*Aspergillus*
    - Parasites—*Toxoplasma*, cryptosporidium, Ascariasis
- Trauma—Abdominal injury
- ERCP
- Congenital—Choledochocoele, Pancreas divisum
- Vascular—Ischaemia, atheroembolism, vasculitis
- Genetic—CFTR and other genetic mutations
- Idiopathic

Gallstones. They are the most common cause of acute pancreatitis accounting for 35–40% of cases. However, only 3–7% of patients with gallstones develop pancreatitis. Small gallstones less than 5 mm in diameter are associated with increased risk of pancreatitis.

Alcohol. It is the second most common cause of acute pancreatitis.

Hypertriglyceridemia. Serum triglyceride concentrations above 1000 mg/dl can precipitate attacks of acute pancreatitis.

Post-ERCP. Acute pancreatitis occurs in about 5% of patients undergoing therapeutic ERCP.

Hypercalcaemia. Hypercalcaemia of any cause can lead to acute pancreatitis.

Genetic mutations. Several genetic mutations have been associated with pancreatitis. Inherited forms of pancreatitis may present as recurrent acute pancreatitis but eventually progress to chronic pancreatitis.

PRSSI, CFTR, SPINK1

Drugs. Pancreatitis due to drugs is rare. Clinical features of drug induced pancreatitis are indistinguishable from acute pancreatitis, hence a high index of suspicion is required.

Prognosis of drug induced pancreatitis is excellent.

Pancreatitis has been associated with infections listed above.

Around 70% of individuals have a characteristic syndrome caused by infections.

Pancreas divisum is present in 7% of people, whether it causes pancreatitis is controversial.

Idiopathic. In more than 15 to 25% of cases no cause is found.

Clinical features. Acute pancreatitis should be suspected in patients with severe acute abdominal pain.

Most patients with acute pancreatitis have acute onset of persistent severe epigastric pain.

In gallstone pancreatitis pain is well-localized and onset of pain is rapid. In other causes, onset of pain is poorly localized and less abrupt. In half the patients pain radiates to back.

Pain persists for several hours to days and may be partially relieved by sitting up or bending forward.

90% of patients have associated nausea and vomiting.

Patients with severe acute pancreatitis may have dyspnoea.

5–10% patients with acute severe pancreatitis may have painless disease and have unexplained hypotension, e.g. post-operative and critically ill-patients.

Patients receiving incriminating drugs may initially be monitored by serum amylase and lipase estimations.

Physical Examination

Physical findings vary depending upon the severity of acute pancreatitis. In patients with mild acute pancreatitis the epigastrium may be minimally tender to palpation. In contrast patient with severe pancreatitis there is significant tenderness. Patients may have abdominal distension and reduced bowel sound due to ileus secondary to inflammation.

Patients with severe pancreatitis may have fever, tachypnoea, hypoglycaemia and hypotension.

In 3% of patients with acute pancreatitis ecchymotic discolouration may be observed in the periumbilical region (Cullen's sign) or along the flank (Grey turner sign). These findings suggest presence of retroperitoneal bleeding.

Investigations

There is leakage of pancreatic enzymes from acinar cells into systemic circulation. Serum amylase rises within 6 to 12 hours of the onset of acute pancreatitis and in uncomplicated attacks returns to normal within 3 to 5 days.

Serum amylase elevation of greater than 3 times normal has a sensitivity of 80% and specificity of 90%. Serum amylase elevations may not be seen in 20% of cases of alcoholic pancreatitis as well as hyper-triglyceridemia associated pancreatitis.

The diagnosis is missed in the patients who may present more than 24 hours after onset of pancreatitis.

Serum amylase is not specific for acute pancreatitis and may be elevated in the other conditions also like renal failure, cholecystitis, etc.

Serum lipase has a sensitivity and specificity for acute pancreatitis ranging from 80–100%. Lipase elevations occur earlier and last longer, hence are useful in patients who present after 24 hours after the onset of pain. However, non-specific elevations of lipase have also been reported.

Patients with pancreatitis may have an elevated haematocrit due to haemoconcentration.

Metabolic abnormalities like elevated blood urea nitrogen, hypocalcaemia and hypoglycemia may occur.

Acute pancreatitis is associated with raised C-reactive protein.

Imaging

Abdominal ultrasonogrphy—In case of acute pancreatitis, the pancreas appears diffusely enlarged and hypoechoic on ultrasound examination.

Pancreatic fluid appears anechoic.

Bowel gas due to ileus may prevent sonographic evaluation in 25–35% of cases of acute pancreatitis.

Ultrasound cannot identify necrosis within pancreas.

Abdominal CT Scan

Contrast enhanced abdominal CT Scan shows focal or diffuse enlargement with heterogenous enhancement suggestive of acute edematous pancreatitis.

Necrosis of pancreatic tissue is recognized as lack of enhancement after IV contrast.

CT scan performed three days after the onset of acute pancreatitis establishes the presence and extent of pancreatic necrosis and local complications.

It may also pick-up CBD stone or pancreatic mass if present.

MRI Scan. On MRI T1 weighted images with fat suppression, diffuse or focal enlargement of the pancreatic gland can be seen in acute pancreatitis. The margins of pancreas are blurred.

Acute Pancreatitis is divided into

1. Mild acute pancreatitis which is characterized by absence of organ failure and local or systemic complications.
2. Moderately severe acute pancreatitis which is characterized by transient organ failure (resolves within 48 hours) and or local or systemic complications without persistent organ failure.
3. Severe acute pancreatitis is characterized by persistent organ failure.

The diagnosis of acute pancreatitis requires the presence of two of the following three criteria:
1. Acute onset of persistent, severe, epigastric pain often radiating to back

2. Elevation in serum amylase or lipase to three times greater than upper limit of normal
3. Characteristic findings of acute pancreatitis on imaging (CT or MRI or abdominal ultrasound).

In patients in whom diagnosis is uncertain CT scan of abdomen is done to exclude other causes of abdominal pain. In patients with renal failure, an abdominal MRI is preferred.

Differential Diagnosis

- Peptic ulcer disease
- Choledocholithiasis or cholangitis
- Cholecystitis
- Perforated viscus
- Intestinal obstruction
- Mesenteric ischaemia
- Hepatitis

Once the diagnosis of acute pancreatitis is established, aetiology is to be determined.

History should include previous symptoms or documentation of gallstones, alcohol, history of hypertriglyceridemia or hypercalcemia, family history of pancreatic disease, drug history, history of trauma and autoimmune disease.

Investigations include serum amylase and lipase, S. triglyceride, S. calcium, liver biochemistry, pancreatic imaging with sonography for cholelithiasis and choledocholithiasis.

CT scan is carried out to evaluate pancreatic morphology, presence of complications and to rule out underlying malignancy if any.

Endoscopic ultrasound is indicated for small pancreatic cancer, ampullary masses, features of chronic pancreatitis and microlithiasis.

Management of Acute Pancreatitis

Assessment of Disease Severity

At initial evaluation the severity of acute pancreatitis should be assessed for fluid losses and organ failure.

Serial measurements of amylase and lipase are not useful to predict disease severity or prognosis.

Abdominal CT scan is to be done after 72 hours to see complete extent of pancreatic and peripancreatic necrosis. It may be done earlier if there is diagnostic uncertainty.

Patients with severe acute pancreatitis with organ failure or haemodynamic instability require to be admitted to an intensive care unit.

Initial management of patients with acute pancreatitis consists of fluid resuscitation, pain control and nutritional support.

Fluid Replacement

Aggressive hydration at 5 to 10 ml/kg/hour of crystalloid, e.g. normal saline is necessary unless patient has cardiovascular, renal or other comorbid factors. Fluid requirements should be reassessed at frequent intervals up to 48 hours. The rate of fluid resuscitation should be adjusted based on clinical assessment, haematocrit and blood urea nitrogen (BUN) values.

Increased fluid resuscitation should be considered in patients whose BUN levels do not fall. Continued aggressive fluid resuscitation is not advisable beyond 48 hours.

Pain control. Uncontrolled pain can contribute to haemodynamic instability. Opioids are the drugs of choice. Fentanyl is increasingly used.

Patients with acute pancreatitis should be monitored closely in first 48 hours for organ failure.

Nutrition. Patients with mild pancreatitis can be managed with intravenous hydration alone. Patients with moderately severe or severe pancreatitis require nutritional support.

In mild pancreatitis, oral feeding can be started after 48 hours when pain subsides. In severe pancreatitis oral feeding is not tolerated due to postprandial pain, nausea or vomiting. Patients usually require enteral or parenteral feeding.

Enteral feeding is preferred over parenteral feeding. Enteral feeding requires placement of a jejunal feeding tube. Enteral nutrition helps to maintain the intestinal barrier and prevents bacterial translocation from gut. Parenteral nutrition should be initiated in patients who do not tolerate enteral feeding.

Antibiotics

Up to 20 % of patients with acute pancreatitis develop an extra pancreatic infection and require antibiotics.

Prophylactic antibiotics are not recommended.

Complications

Local complications of acute pancreatitis include acute peripancreatic fluid collections, pancreatic pseudocyst, acute necrotic collection and walled off necrosis.

Acute peripancreatic fluid collections develop in early phase of pancreatitis, they remain asymptomatic and resolve spontaneously.

Infected Necrosis

Occurrence of pancreatic infection is a leading cause of morbidity and mortality in acute necrotizing pancreatitis. One-third of patients of pancreatic necrosis develop infection. It is commonly seen after 10 days. The majority are monomicrobial gut derived organism, e.g. E. Coli, Enterococci. Infected necrosis should be suspected in patients with pancreatitis who deteriorate.

Empiric antibiotics are initiated with antibiotics known to penetrate pancreatic necrosis, e.g. carbapenem.

In stable patients with infected necrosis attempt is made to delay necrosectomy by continuing antibiotics for 4 weeks.

Necrosectomy should be done by endoscopic or percutaneous radiologic approach. If it is not possible or fails open surgical necrosectomy is to be done.

Sterile necrosis is to be managed conservatively but occasionally may require intervention if symptomatic.

Peripancreatic Vascular Complications

Splanchnic venous thrombosis, thrombosis of splenic, portal or superior mesenteric veins is seen in 1 to 24 % of patients. treatment is supportive unless there is extension of thrombus.

Pseudoaneurysms are rare but should be suspected when patients with acute pancreatitis have unexplained gastrointestinal bleeding or sudden expansion of pancreatic fluid collection. Treatment is by angiographic embolisation.

Management of Underlying Conditions

Gallstone Pancreatitis

Most stones pass into duodenum and require no immediate intervention.

If stones obstruct the biliary duct or ampulla of vater, it can cause acute pancreatitis with cholangitis. In this case emergency ERCP with papillotomy is to be performed in 24 hours. If there is no cholangitis ERCP may be deferred.

All patients with mild pancreatitis, cholecystectomy is to be done preferably during the same hospitalization. In severe necrotizing pancreatitis cholecystectomy is to be done when inflammation subsides and fluid collections resolve or stabilize.

20

Chronic Pancreatitis

Viral Patrawala

Chronic pancreatitis is a syndrome involving inflammatory changes in the pancreas that result in a permanent structural damage which can lead to impairment of exocrine and endocrine functiocns.

Aetiology

- Alcohol abuse
- Ductal obstruction due to trauma, pseudo-cysts, stones, tumours
- Tropical pancreatitis
- Idiopathic pancreatitis
- Autoimmune pancreatitis
- Genetic causes (mutations in cystic fibrosis gene, hereditary pancreatitis).

Clinical Manifestations

The two primary clinical manifestations of chronic pancreatitis are abdominal pain and pancreatic insufficiency.

Abdominal pain is present in 80 to 95% of patients. Pain is typically epigastric and radiates to back, pain may occur 15 to 30 minutes after food and may be relieved by sitting up and bending forward.

Pancreatic insufficiency develops when 90% of pancreatic function is lost.

Steatorrhoea occurs prior to protein deficiency as lipolytic activity decreases earlier than proteolysis. Patient has loose greasy, foul smelling, stools which are difficult to flush. Malabsorption of fat soluble vitamins A, D, E, K and vitamin B12 may occur.

Pancreatic Diabetes

Diabetes occurs late in the course of disease and is more common in patients with chronic calcifying disease. Diabetes usually requires insulin replacement but as glucagon producing cells are also lost hypoglycaemia is more common.

Complications of Chronic Pancreatitis

- Pseudocyst formation
- Bile duct or duodenal obstruction
- Pancreatic ascites
- Splenic vein thrombosis, pseudoaneruysm
- Pancreatic cancer.

Diagnosis

The diagnosis of chronic pancreatitis is challenging as laboratory studies and imaging procedures may be normal. The triad of pancreatic calcifications, steatorrhoea and diabetes mellitus occurs late in the disease.

Laboratory Studies

Serum concentrations of amylase and lipase may be slightly elevated but are more commonly normal.

Complete blood count and liver function tests are normal.

Fecal elastase and 72 hours fecal fat are helpful for evaluating pancreatic exocrine dysfunction.

Imaging Studies

Transabdominal sonography has sensitivity of 60–70% specificity of 80–90%. It shows bulky pancreas, calcification, dilated irregular pancreatic duct. It may also reveal complications like pseudocyst.

CT scanning has sensitivity of 75–90% and specificity of 85%.

MRCP is the diagnostic test of choice since it can demonstrate calcification and pancreatic duct obstruction.

Endoscopic ultrasound:

The most predictive feature is the presence of stones.

The other features are visible side branches, czysts, lobularity, dilatation of main pancreatic duct, irregular main pancreatic duct.

Treatment

Treatment of chronic pancreatitis is treatment of symptoms.

- Pain management
- Cessation of alcohol intake
- Small meals and hydration
- Supplementation with medium chain triglycerides may help
- Cessation of smoking.

Pancreatic Enzymes Supplements

Lipase requirement is of around 30000 IU with every meal.

Analgesics are used if pancreatic enzyme therapy levels fails. Amitriptyline may help.

Chronic opoid analgesia may be required in patients with persistent pain.

Adjuvant therapy with pregabalin is helpful.

Antioxidant therapy may help.

Specialized Approach

Coeliac nerve block is performed percutaneously or endoscopically with alcohol or steroids. It has limited success. Symptoms frequently relapse in 2 to 6 months.

Endoscopic Therapy

Endoscopic therapy is aimed at decompressing an obstructed pancreatic duct. It helps in pain relief. Endoscopic treatment is done in patients who have a dominant stricture or stone obstructing in the head.

Surgery is considered for patients who do not respond to medical therapy.

Surgery is either drainage procedures or pancreatic resection.

Decompression procedures are for patients with refractory pain and a dilated main pancreatic duct. The dilated pancreatic duct is anastomosed to a loop of duodenum.

Short-term pain relief is present in approximately 80% of patients.

Resection usually involves resection of a part of the pancreas usually the head, less commonly the entire pancreas.

Treatment of Steatorrhoea

- Dietary modification
- Fat restrictions to 20 gm per day
- Lipase supplementation 30,000 IU/meal
- Vitamin supplementation, fat soluble vitamin deficiency is common. Vitamin D supplementation is required.
- Medium chain triglycerides are helpful in patients not responding to diet and pancreatic enzyme supplementation.

Management of endocrine dysfunction: Calcific pancreatitis is complicated by hyperglycaemia due to insulin deficiency caused by loss of beta cells. Blood sugar levels fluctuate due to erratic food intake, malabsorption, intrinsic insulin secretion. It is better managed with insulin therapy.

21

Ca Pancreas

Prabha Sawant, Nirav Pipaliya

INTRODUCTION

Pancreatic cancer is one of our most lethal malignancies. Despite substantial improvements in the survival rates for other major cancer forms, pancreatic cancer survival rates have remained relatively unchanged since the 1960s. Pancreatic cancer is usually detected at an advanced stage and most treatment regimens are ineffective, contributing to the poor overall prognosis. Up to 20% of patients are eligible for initial resection. Even after potential curative resection, most patients will eventually have recurrence, and 5-year survival of completely resected patients is only up to 25%.

EPIDEMIOLOGY

American Cancer Society reported that pancreatic cancer had surpassed breast cancer as the third leading cause of cancer related death in the United States. The global annual incidence rate for pancreas cancer is about 8/100,000 persons. Worldwide, pancreatic cancer accounts for more than 200000 deaths every year. Total deaths from pancreatic cancer are currently increasing and are predicted to be the second leading cause of cancer death in the USA by 2030. Incidence is lowest among populations in India, Africa, and Southeast Asia, but under diagnosis in regions with poorer access to care might bias these estimates. In India, the annual incidence of pancreatic cancer is 0.5–2.4 per 100,000 men and 0.2–1.8 per 100,000 women. Incidence is slightly higher in urban male population of western and northern India. The incidence of pancreatic cancer also differs between the sexes: incidence is 50% higher in men than in women. Pancreatic cancer is a disease of older adults, with most cases occurring in patients between 60 and 80 years of age.

Risk Factors

The risk factors and established genetic syndromes associated with pancreatic adenocarcinoma are shown in Tables 21.1 and 21.2, respectively. Although it is estimated that 5 to 10% of pancreatic cancers have an inherited component, the genetic basis for familial aggregation has not been identified in most cases. Among people with a known family history of pancreatic cancer in a first-degree relative, as compared with the general population, the relative risk of the development of pancreatic cancer is increased by a factor

Table 21.1: Risk factors

- Smoking
- Chronic pancreatitis
- Diabetes mellitus
- Obesity
- Non-O blood group
- Chlorinated hydrocarbons

Table 21.2: Hereditary syndromes associated with pancreatic cancer

Syndrome	Gene	Chromosome
• Hereditary pancreatitis	PRSS1, SPINK1	7, 5
• Peutz-Jeghers syndrome	STK11 [LKB1]	19
• Familial atypical multiple mole and melanoma syndrome	CDKN2A (P16)	9
• Hereditary breast and ovarian cancer syndromes	BRCA2	13
• Hereditary non-polyposis colon cancer (Lynch syndrome)	MLH1, MSH2, MSH6	Multiple
• Familial pancreatic cancer (monoallelic)	ATM	11

of 2, 6 and 30 in people with one, two, and three affected family members, respectively.

The most well-established risk factor for pancreatic cancer is cigarette smoking, causing a 75% increased risk that persists at least 10 years after smoking cessation. Chronic pancreatitis of any cause substantially increases lifetime risk of pancreatic cancer. Patients with diabetes, both type I and II, have a 30% excess risk of pancreatic cancer, which persists for more than 20 years after initial diagnosis of diabetes, suggesting that diabetes is not merely a marker of pancreatic dysfunction as a result of neoplasia. It is difficult to implicate alcohol as an independent risk factor for pancreatic cancer because of the close association between alcohol and smoking—a proven risk factor for pancreatic cancer. If alcohol affects pathogenesis of pancreatitis, it could promote the effects of other risk factors, such as smoking. Recent studies concluded that heavy drinkers might have an increased risk of pancreatic cancer.

Pathophysiology

The majority (95%) of pancreatic cancers develop as adenocarcinomas from the ductal cells of the exocrine pancreas. Of them 1% is of acinar origin, 1% is of non-epithelial origin and 3% are of uncertain cellular origin. It is associated with an accumulation of mutations with progressive morphological changes. The current model proposes a progression from normal cuboidal to low columnar epithelium

through a series of lesions termed pancreatic intraepithelial neoplasia (PanIN) to invasive carcinoma. Pancreatic cancer can also arise from intraductal papillary mucinous neoplasms (IPMN) and mucinous cystic neoplasms (MCN). Various genes mutations found in pancreatic cancer are shown in Table 21.3.

Presentation

Approximately 60 to 70% of pancreatic cancers are located in the head of the pancreas, and 20 to 25% are located in the body and tail of the pancreas. The presenting signs and symptoms are related to the location. Head tumour presents relatively early due to proximity to the common bile duct with symptoms of obstructive jaundice like icterus, itching and clay stools. Tumours in the body and tail presents late with abdominal pain radiating to back and sometimes, lump. Other

Table 21.3: Gene mutations associated with pancreatic cancer

Gene mutation	Incidence (%)
K-ras 2	95
P16/CDKN2A	80
P21	75–85
TP53	50–75
Cyclin D1	95
DPC4/MADH4	55
Telomerase	95
BRCA-2	7–10
LKB1/STK11, MKK4, TGFb1/11, RB1	5

common symptoms are weight loss, asthenia, and anorexia. Diabetes is present in at least 50% of patients with pancreatic cancer. Weight loss can arise from anorexia, maldigestion from pancreatic ductal obstruction, and cachexia. Occasionally, pancreatic-duct obstruction could result in attacks of pancreatitis. Deep and superficial venous thrombosis (Trousseau's sign) might be a presenting sign. Gastric-outlet obstruction with nausea and vomiting is a manifestation of more advanced disease. Less common manifestations include panniculitis and depression. About 25% of patients with pancreatic cancer have diabetes mellitus at diagnosis and another 40% have impaired glucose tolerance. The cause of the diabetogenic state is uncertain, but diabetes is sometimes cured by resection of pancreatic cancer. Researchers are investigating whether early-stage pancreatic cancer should be looked for in older individuals with new-onset diabetes.

Diagnosis and Staging

Ultrasonography (USG)

USG is generally initial modality used in a patient presented with obstructive jaundice. It is used to confirm biliary dilatation and cholelithiasis. Pancreatic mass may be missed on USG.

Computed Tomography (CT)

Tri-phasic pancreatic-protocol CT is the gold standard diagnostic test for pancreatic cancer. It is also best for disease staging. The pancreatic CT protocol consists of dual-phase scanning using IV and oral contrast agents. The first, arterial (pancreatic) phase is obtained 40 seconds after administration of IV contrast agent. At this time maximum enhancement of the normal pancreas is obtained, allowing identification of non-enhancing neoplastic lesions. The second, portalvenous phase is obtained 70 seconds after injection of IV contrast agent and allows accurate detection of liver metastases and

assessment of tumour involvement of the portal and mesenteric veins. Overall sensitivity of CT for pancreatic cancer is 86% to 97%, but sensitivity for lesions less than 2 cm is near 77%.

CT criteria for unresectability of a pancreatic tumour are distant metastasis (e.g. to liver, peritoneum, or other sites), encasement of the celiac axis orsuperior mesenteric artery, and/ or occlusion of the portal vein or superior mesenteric vein. Using these criteria, CT has been shown to be almost 100% accurate in predicting unresectable disease. However, some patients (5% to 15%) predicted to have resectable disease according to these CT criteria are found at laparoscopy to have unresectable lesions.

Endoscopic Ultrasound (EUS)

Strengths of EUS as a staging tool are its ability to image small pancreatic tumours especially less than 2 cm in size and ability to acquire a tissue sample by FNA to provide a histological diagnosis. There are, however, some inherent limitations of EUS in local staging of pancreas cancer. The imaging by EUS, unlike CT, isoperator dependent. The ability of EUS to accurately detect loco regional invasion or encasement of vessels other than the portal vein is limited. EUS also cannot detect distal metastasis. EUS is unlikely to change surgical decision-making in the patient presenting with typical findings who is resectable by CT criteria. EUS FNA is necessary when some other tumour type (e.g. Lymphoma, neuroendocrine tumour) is suspected. It is also helpful to arrive at the histological diagnosis before embarking on palliative or neoadjuvant chemotherapy.

PET-CT

Positron emission tomography (PET) CT scan has no much role in the diagnosis of pancreatic cancer. However, it may be useful in assessing tumour recurrence after pancreatic resection, when scar tissue or post-operative changes

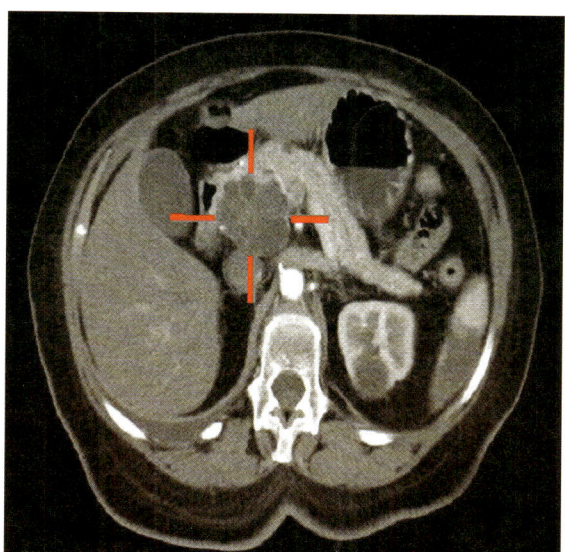

Fig. 21.1: A computed tomography (CT) scan showing a hypodense mass lesion in the head of the pancreas, most likely pancreatic cancer

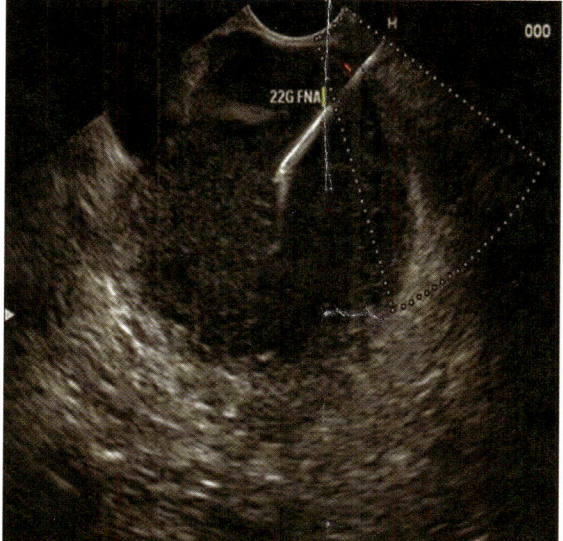

Fig. 21.2: An Endoscopic ultrasound (EUS) image showing a hypoechoic mass lesion with a FNA needle inside the lesion

may be difficult to differentiate from recurrent carcinoma. PET/CT can also be of benefit in assessing tumour response to primary or neoadjuvant chemotherapy, which may lead to alteration in clinical management.

CA 19-9

Tumour marker CA 19-9 aids in diagnosis, prognosis and response to treatment. Serum level more than 37 IL/ml has a sensitivity and specificity of 86% and 87%, respectively, to diagnose pancreatic cancer. Preoperative CA19-9 of more than 100–200 U/mL predict unresectability and poor survival. Patients with post-operative levels above 90 U/mL do not benefit from adjuvant chemotherapy.

Laparoscopy

Existing radiographic staging modalities are inaccurate at detecting low-volume small peritoneal implants and small surface liver metastasis. Laparoscopy is advocated for all patients with tumours in the body and tail of the pancreas (in which the frequency of unsuspected metastases approaches 50%) and for patients with tumours larger than 2 cm in the head of the pancreas, because the yield of laparoscopy is proportional to the size of the primary tumour.

Staging

The American Joint Committee on Cancer (AJCC) staging system for pancreatic cancer is shown in Table 21.4.

Treatment

Patients with pancreatic cancer are best managed by a multidisciplinary team that includes oncologists, surgeons, radiologists, gastroenterologists, pathologists, pain management experts, dietitians and palliative care experts.

General Principles

Pancreatic cancer, at presentation, are categorized as resectable, borderline resectable, or Unresectable (locally advanced or metastatic) on the basis of vascular invasion and distal metastasis (Table 21.5). Resectable and borderline resectable cancers are typically stage I or II cancers; unresectable tumour saregenerally stage III or IV. Patient with resectable disease are treated with surgery.

Table 21.4: The American Joint Committee on Cancer (AJCC) staging system for pancreatic cancer

Tumour (T)

TX: Primary tumour cannot be assessed

T0: No evidence of primary tumour

Tis: Carcinoma *in situ* (includes grade III pancreatic intraepithelial neoplasia [PanIN])

T1: Tumour limited to the pancreas, ≤2 cm in greatest dimension

T2: Tumour limited to the pancreas, >2 cm in greatest dimension

T3: Tumour extends beyond the pancreas but without involvement of the celiac axis or the superior mesenteric artery

T4: Tumorinvolves celiac axis or superior mesenteric artery (unresectable primary tumour)

Lymph Node Metastases (N)

NX: Regional lymph nodes cannot be assessed

N0: No regional lymph node metastasis

N1: Regional lymph node metastasis

Distant Metastases (M)

MX: Distant metastasis cannot be assessed

M0: No distant metastasis

M1: Distant metastasis

AJCC Staging

Stage 0   : Tis N0 M0

Stage IA : T1 N0 M0

Stage IB : T2 N0 M0

Stage IIA : T3 N0 M0

Stage IIB : T1 N1 M0

                 T2 N1 M0

                 T3 N1 M0

Stage III : T4 N1 M0

Stage IV : Any T Any N M1

Borderline resectable tumours are offered neoadjuvant chemotherapy or chemoradiation with a goal of reducing disease burden and perhaps with an eye toward resection in the future. Patients with unresectable metastatic tumors are typically offered chemotherapy as a palliativetreatment approach. Chemoradiotherapy downstages about 30% of patients with locally advanced disease to resectable pancreatic cancer, and these individuals go on to achieve median survival similar to that for those who have initially resectable disease.

Surgery

Surgical resection is the only potentially curative treatment for pancreatic cancer. Because of advanced disease at presentation, only about 15% to 20% of patients are candidates for surgery. The most common operation for pancreatic cancer is Whipple's pancreaticoduodenectomy (Fig. 21.3), which removes primarily the head of the pancreas en bloc withthe duodenum, distal bile duct, and proximal jejunum, with pancreaticojejunal anastomosis. Operative mortality is less than 3%. In view of high incidence of complications, preoperative biliary drainage is usually not recommended unless patient has cholangitis, surgery is delayed or neoadjuvant chemotherapy is planned. Distal pancreatectomy is performed forcancers of the body or tail with an en bloc splenectomy for a more comprehensive lymphadenectomy. Five-year survival rates even after resection remain approximately 25% only.

Table 21.5: Criteria defining resectability status

Resectablity status	Arterial involvement	Venous contact
Resectable	No any arterial contact	No contact or contact up to 180° With superior mesenteric vein (SMV) or portal vein (PV)
Borderline	Head tumour: Contact with common hepatic Artery (CHA) without extension to celiac artery (CA) OR contact with SMA <180° Body/tail tumour: Contact with CA < 180°	Contact of >180° with SMV/PV or Any contact with IVC
Unresectable	Metastasis (including non-regional lymph nodes) or contact with SMA/CA> 180°	Unreconstructible PV/SMV due to tumour thrombus

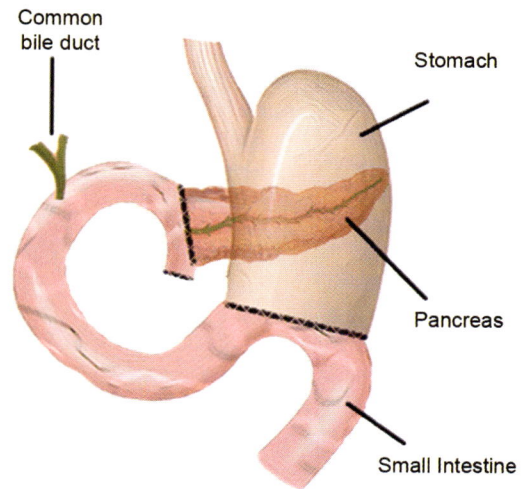

Common bile duct

Stomach

Pancreas

Small Intestine

Fig. 21.3: A schematic diagram depicting Whipple's pancreaticoduodenectomy surgery

and tumour size more than 2.5 cm. Currently, gemcitabine based therapy is recommended. Role of radiotherapy as adjuvant treatment is doubtful.

Neoadjuvant Treatment

Neoadjuvant therapy is defined as treatment given prior to surgery in order to reduce disease burden. It has the potential to downstage patients with borderline resectable disease to facilitate resection and it is usually recommended in this setting only. Tumour response rates to current neoadjuvant therapies are not high, and delaying surgical resection could also allow disease progression. For this reason, patients undergoing neoadjuvant therapy should be restaged before surgical resection.

Adjuvant Treatment

Adjuvant therapy is defined as treatment given after surgery to prevent cancer recurrence. Adjuvant treatment is recommended for individuals who undergo pancreatic resection with curative intent especially in patients with high chances of recurrence. Risk factors for recurrent disease include positive margins, lymph node involvement, high-grade tumours,

Palliative Treatment

For distant metastatic disease, current recommendation is to give combination therapy with either FOLFIRINOX (folinic acid, fluorouracil, irinotecan, oxaliplatin) or with gemcitabine plus nab-paclitaxel for those patients with a good performance status who can tolerate combination therapy or gemcitabine alone for those who cannot.

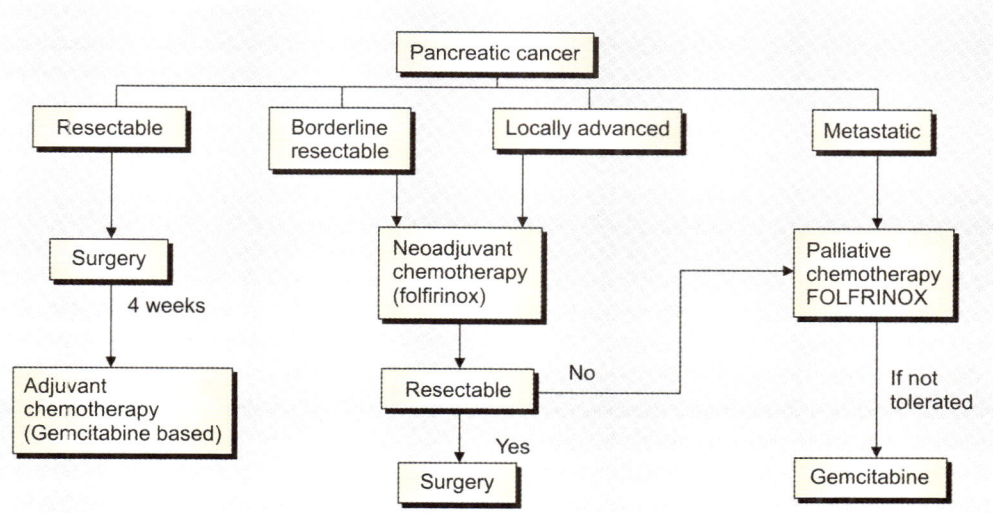

Fig. 21.4: Simplified management algorithm for pancreatic cancer

For palliation of jaundice, endoscopic biliary metallic or plastic stenting is advocated. Endoscopic drainage is superior to surgical drainage in terms of low morbidity and mortality of the procedure. For pain relief, WHO pain ladder protocol is followed. EUS guided celiac ganglion neurolysis is performed for intractable pain.

For symptoms of gastric outlet obstruction, surgical gastrojejunostomy or endoscopic duodenal metallic stenting can be performed.

General Approach to Management

Overall approach to the management is shown in Fig. 21.4.

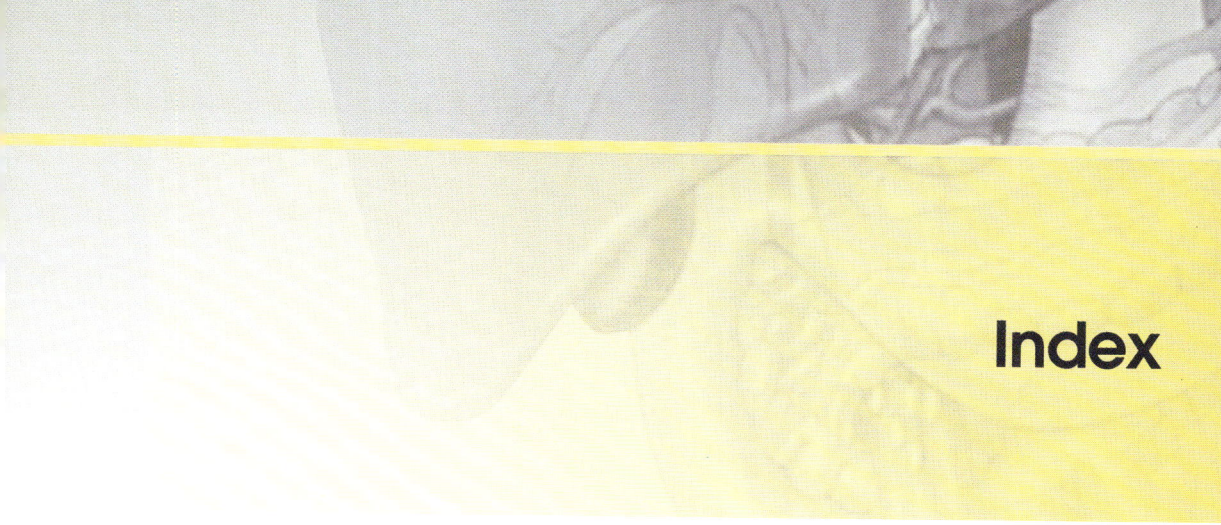

Index